HOW TO MAKE PEACE WITH FOOD

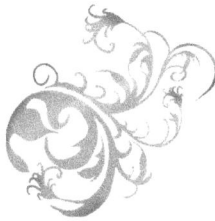

Rediscover your personal power of choice

Sandra Yelich, MSW

Published by CYK Publishing
Cover art by CC Covers

What people are saying about
How to Make Peace with Food

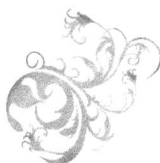

"I was unhappy about my looks and my weight. I felt out of control. **Now I can accept my body**, yet know that I have the power to change it in a comfortable, realistic, in-control fashion."

"I was so embarrassed and guilty about my eating. **Now my bingeing has stopped.** This has been more in-depth than I expected."

"I now have the **confidence** to eat the way I really want to."

"I had a negative image of my body, appearance, and weight. **Now I understand why I eat** and I can stop and listen to my body to see if I'm really hungry."

"After this program, I feel pretty damn good. **Mirrors are no longer my enemy.**"

"I was out of control with my eating. **Now I know I am in control** of my life."

Acknowledgments

I have had a lot of help along the way to creating this program and I'd like to acknowledge those who have been generous with their time and teaching.

I'd like to acknowledge Lois Rollman and her non-diet support group for getting me started on this path, Jane Hirschman and Carol Munter for some wonderful non-diet ideas as set forth in their book <u>Overcoming Overeating</u>, and workshop presenters everywhere for the experience that led to the creation of this program.

I also appreciate all the struggles, sharing, insights, and feedback from everyone who has gone through this program as well. You've helped make it what it is today.

Thanks to all of you.

TABLE OF CONTENTS

INTRODUCTION

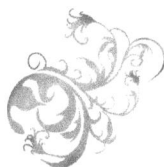

How To Make Peace With Food

The Difference

Welcome!

You are reading a book about food and eating that is more than the same tired material about diets and weight-loss, with which you are probably already familiar. *How To Make Peace With Food* is a series of informational and experiential sessions that help you examine your un-healthy and destructive beliefs of what food and eating mean to you in a way that enables you to make and maintain the changes you have wanted, but have felt incapable of accomplishing.

How To Make Peace With Food is <u>not</u> a diet or weight-loss program, nor is it a quick-fix solution to the problem of out-of-control or unhealthy eating. Instead, it is a way of learning how to **eat to live** instead of repeatedly **living** (and dying) **to eat**. It's educational and holistic in its scope, *proceeding beyond counting calories to provide you with the means of counting on yourself.*

How To Make Peace With Food helps you understand some of the basis and rationale for your non-natural eating patterns, gives you new information as to why you may be stuck in the lose/gain cycle of dieting, and encourages you through weekly assignments to explore, in-depth, those eating patterns that continue to keep you trapped. It gives you new options for making the transition from destructive eating patterns and choices to the more natural patterns that fit best with your body, as well as insight as to why and how you may have sabotaged your progress in the past, so that you can avoid similar pitfalls in the future.

How To Make Peace With Food was originally set up for weekly group participation. Within the six weeks of the program, group members began making changes: self-esteem and self-acceptance rose, negative thinking about themselves lessened, eating patterns and food choices improved, and perceptions and perspectives about why they have been struggling transformed. This was the beginning of restoring their body's weight to a weight that was more natural and healthier for them as individuals.

This book is an attempt to recreate as much as possible the experience of the weekly classes in written form. It includes the answers to many of the questions that have been asked within the context of the groups. It also includes the contents of the group's workbook and the weekly homework assignments.

While you won't be able to share the same involvement as those participants who actually attend the program in a group format, you will be able to get valuable information from this book regarding your own non-natural eating patterns and self-destructive choices. It is recommended that you read one chapter at a time, complete the assignment, then allow at least a week before moving to the next chapter. It's also important to remember to go at your own pace. This is your individual process.

This interim week gives you the chance to process and integrate the information from each chapter into your daily routine. This is an active, dynamic program, designed to be <u>used</u>, not just read. It is in utilizing the information on a day-to-day basis that change can happen. After all, you are currently practicing your present eating patterns daily. The only way to make the changes you want is to begin practicing something new to take their place.

The assignments are for you. Through them you will be able to explore aspects of yourself and your eating in ways you may not have considered before. There are no right or wrong ways to do the assignments, but each affords you with information and insight into the why's and wherefores of your own patterns and choices.

This program is meant to be informational and educational only. It is not designed to take the place of therapy, and cannot be held responsible for decisions by the reader. Although there may be therapeutic issues that are revealed to you along the way, *I cannot recommend strongly enough that if an emotional crisis presents itself to you, seek professional help.* Often there are buried issues that you may or may not have been aware of that have fueled your destructive eating patterns. A professional counselor or therapist can assist you in working through anything that becomes too uncomfortable or overwhelming.

How To Make Peace With Food will give you a foundation for changing and maintaining healthier and more personal food and eating choices. You will receive information and insights which will help you distinguish between natural and non-natural messages about food and eating, how to listen to and respect them, and how to use the information you gain to re-establish control of your eating.

This program is not directed toward goals of size and weight. It focuses on health and happiness for your life. It's not for everyone. However, if you are tired of constantly struggling with dieting, battling with yourself to eat "right" and don't know what else to do, **_How To Make Peace With Food_** may be what you've been looking for.

CHAPTER I

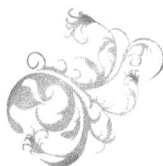

ACCEPTING OURSELVES

The Battle Rages On

So many of us struggle with food. On one hand we love the way it smells and tastes and we love to eat it; on the other hand, we hate how much we love it and what loving it does to us. We feel trapped. Just when the problem seems in hand and we believe we are finally managing everything nicely, something happens to cause us to slip and sabotage our success. Soon we feel totally out of control again. Some of us have all but given up in a frustrated sense of hopelessness.

Not knowing what to do next, we try every new diet that comes along. We're sure that happiness will be ours if we just win the battle with our weight. Unfortunately, the perfect diet is non-existent. After losing all that "ugly fat" and loving ourselves for having this wonderful new body, the weight starts creeping back. We begin hating ourselves once again for being weak and out of control. We ask ourselves, "What's wrong with me? Why can't I do what seems to be so easy for others?" The lose/gain cycle comes full circle once again and the frustration with ourselves and our lives returns.

For some people, depression or self-hate increases and turns into a constant companion. For others, a defensive attitude toward diets and weight develops and rebellion sets in. In any case, the frustration can become overwhelming with a sense of hopelessness pervading their lives, resulting in feeling miserable.

We were created to be comfortable and compatible with food. Our bodies transmit the messages we need to enable us to choose which foods and how much of each to put into our bodies. For example, think of how a baby lets someone know when they're hungry, and how that baby will also spit the nipple out when full. That baby is listening to their own body's individual messages and acting accordingly.

You, too, were originally in touch with your body's messages about food and eating. Somewhere along the line, however, your body's natural messages became hidden, ignored, or overridden, and unhealthy messages took their place. Because of this, you may have forgotten how to tell when you're hungry, when you're full, or whether eating is even what your body really wants.

For many of us food has become both our best friend and our worst enemy, which makes eating the site of an emotional battleground. Clothing sizes and scales have become our personal dictators, telling us when to feel good about ourselves and when to feel bad. Our emotions, thoughts, and behaviors frequently become food-centered. We habitually eat or refrain from eating without thinking. The result is that we end up hating ourselves for being weak and out of control and hurting ourselves through destructive eating patterns and food choices.

While you read this book and work this program, you will learn that having a natural, healthy relationship with food eliminates the battle. You will learn how to listen to and respect your body's messages about food and eating. Food will take its rightful place in your life as a nourisher rather than a nurturer. Eating will take its natural place as the means to provide your body with the fuel it needs instead of as a problem solver. You will regain a balance in your life concerning food and eating that enables you to do those things that contribute to your having a happy, healthy, and personally fulfilling life.

Food is Not the Enemy – Weight is Not the Problem

You may be wondering, if food is not the enemy and weight is not the problem, then what is? Why are you trapped in these self-destructive cycles of food and eating choices? Why hasn't anything worked? Could this mean that something is wrong with you?

No -- there's nothing wrong with you. For many people facing the challenge of battling non-natural eating patterns, **the real enemy has been a faulty belief system**. This belief system encourages you to have a distorted view of food and eating. When your belief system is faulty, you use food and eating to do things for which they were never intended.

Unfortunately, since your enemy is usually on a subconscious level, you don't regularly realize it's there. You might consciously believe you love yourself and that you deserve the best, but your choices and actions shed light on what those subconscious beliefs are really saying. Your subconscious belief system drives your conscious choices and actions. It's this underlying belief system that must be changed before new choices and behaviors can be maintained.

If the enemy is a faulty belief system, then **the problem is not knowing how to change it** so that you can eat in a way that respects your body. You may have been trained since you were young to eat according to the standards of others, or to use food as a way to comfort or distract yourself when you're facing an uncomfortable situation or emotion.

This training has encouraged you to become out of touch with your body's messages. You don't know how to listen to your body any more, or how to get out from under those old messages that keep you trapped. You don't know how to change your eating patterns, or may even be afraid to do so once you learn how. After all, you've been eating this way for a long time and these eating patterns have seemingly served you well in the past.

Now, you feel that something needs to change. You want to do something different. You're tired of the battle. The old ways don't work well for you anymore. Now it may finally be time to give up your old beliefs and try something new.

Learning to feed yourself what you *truly* need won't necessarily be easy or comfortable. As you continue with this program, you'll have opportunities to explore the many aspects that have discouraged your ability to listen to, trust, and respect your body's messages. As your understanding increases, you'll discover different options, and find/gain the confidence to choose those that work best for you. Above all, you'll learn how to eat for your life instead of for the next party, the next relationship, or the next emotion.

Where's Your Focus?

When you are not taught how to focus on your body and its messages, you'll spend a lot of frustrated time and negative energy focused on food and eating instead. In turn, this keeps your focus off the internal messages your body sends you. By worrying and thinking about if you're eating too much, eating enough, eating the right food, eating the wrong food, or planning future food binges while berating yourself for the last one, you don't leave much time or energy for enjoying the food you're eating in the present.

In order to start identifying just how far away from your body's natural messages your own focus is, turn to the Appendix, Page (i), entitled "Where's Your Focus?" Read through the list of statements. Check off all the statements that pertain to you.

After you've finished that, take a closer look. The more statements you checked off, the more your core belief system dictates that weight is a determining factor for your sense of happiness. Your belief system may have told you that if everything on the outside is perfect, you will be happy, you will be loved, you will not be alone, people will like you and want to be around you, you will have the career you want, or your life will be wonderful. What this means is, you have been focused on other peoples' messages and standards and have ignored what your body says to you. You have been looking for something outside yourself to make you feel happy within.

Learning to be happy from within means bringing the focus *into* yourself. Calories, pounds gained or lost, weight, size, ideal weight standards, body measurements—all these take your focus off what your body is telling you, because your focus is outside yourself. When you are negatively focused on your weight and body image, you are unable to listen to and respect the food and eating messages your body sends you. You may end up confused about why you can't do this right, and why you're so miserable most of the time. You end up judging yourself negatively as a person because you can't control your eating, your food choices, your weight, etc.

Judgments and Acceptance

A negative focus on weight, body image, and fat is generally made up of judgments. These judgments can keep you trapped in a place where the only time you are allowed to feel good about yourself is if you measure up to some outside standard. For instance, if your feelings of happiness depend on being a certain weight, a size two, or having a 20" waistline, you only allow yourself to enjoy your life when these numbers are reached. Any deviation from these numbers can quickly send you into the depths of despair. When you think about it, that doesn't leave a lot of time for feelings of happiness.

What's disturbing for our lives is that most of us find ourselves outside this narrow corridor of happiness much of the time. When we are different from the goal numbers we or others have determined for us, we find ourselves unhappy -- with our weight, with our bodies, with ourselves, with our lives -- and we hate ourselves for our unhappiness. We spend a lot of time in the "if only's" –

- "If only I didn't like chocolate (ice cream, junk food) so much, ...",
- "If only I didn't like to bake, ...",
- "If only I could control myself, ..."
- "If only I weren't so weak, ..."
- "If only I wasn't married, didn't have to cook for my kids, didn't have to go to parties, didn't love eating, etc., I wouldn't have this problem."

In other words, we spend a lot of time and energy blaming ourselves and circumstances for what we perceive to be our own ineffectiveness and lack of willpower when it comes to diets and losing weight.

By negatively judging ourselves we become accustomed to living with the pain of failure. In turn, we transfer these negative judgments about how we look into judgments about ourselves as people. When we fail at a diet, we view ourselves to be failures as people. When you believe that your size, shape, or weight determines what kind of person you are, anything less than perfect means you are a bad person. If size 14 is bad, then you must be bad for being that size. If being fat is bad, and you have decided you are fat, then...well, you get the picture.

This form of logic encourages the judgment of *how* you are to become a judgment of *who* you are. These judgments about fat and how you see yourself in relation to fat set up a negative personal environment around you. Trying to learn, grow, and change in a positive way when surrounded by such negativity can be extremely difficult, if not impossible.

Picture a child in your care. What is the best environment to help that child learn, grow, and change? Is it one of name-calling, put-downs, or ridicule? Or, rather, is it one of acceptance, patience, tolerance for mistakes, and kindness?

The same goes for you. The more negativity you feel about you, the less chance you have for positive growth and learning. If you feel negative about yourself, chances are you will invest very little time, patience, and caring toward your own progress and process. This cultivates a terrain contradictory to change. It contributes to the dynamic of doing the same thing over and over that ends up in shame, guilt, and self-hatred.

The opposite of such negative judgments is acceptance. Most of us have had minimal experience with true acceptance. We usually received messages of acceptance for what we did rather than for who we were. For example, we were judged to be good children if we cleaned our plates. We were judged as bad if we were full and wanted to leave some food behind.

The result of this is that if we didn't *do* something good enough then we were judged not to *be* good enough as people. Transferring these judgments from doing to being became automatic. We stopped focusing on ourselves as unique individuals deserving care and affection no matter what, and began looking for accomplishments and failures as the indication of what kind of people we were and the treatment we deserved.

A personal experience from my childhood shows you what I mean. I always got "A's" and "B's" in school, yet every time I brought a report card home, my dad told me "Well, that's good but next time maybe you can get all A's." As a child, I heard the message that I must get all "A's" in order to get acceptance. With a child's logic, I translated that to mean that I as a person must also be perfect in order to receive any kind of acceptance from someone I loved. While he might have been trying to encourage me to improve, in effect I heard my dad tell me that I wasn't good enough the way I was.

These types of messages may have been repeated to you over and over in many different ways. While the intent may have been thought of as positive by the adult, as a child, your logic resulted in the belief that since you consistently fell short of perfection, you mustn't feel happy until you achieve it. When you incorporated this belief into your day-to-day way of thinking, you've either kept trying to live up to unrealistic ideals and images or you gave up trying at all. You may have even resigned yourself to the idea that it'll never get any better. It is through this type of resignation that acceptance takes on a negative meaning.

Accepting your body or yourself does not mean you are resigned to the way you are and are ready to give up trying to change. On the contrary; accepting yourself means that no matter what you look like, you are not only worth your own love and care, but you are also worth the time and energy needed to make the changes necessary for more personal eating patterns and healthier food choices.

Accepting yourself and your body means acknowledging the reality of your situation. Acceptance encourages you to realize how you have been harming yourself and to learn what is healthy and more natural for you as an individual. It means that you will have patience with yourself for being human and making mistakes. It means a willingness to begin making the changes necessary to keep your body's health and well-being as your primary focus.

In effect, when you don't accept yourself for who you are and how you look, you reject and abandon yourself in many ways:

- You reject the whole reality of who you are by focusing on your weaknesses and overlooking your strengths.
- You see yourself as two-dimensional and forget that you are more than your mistakes or accomplishments.
- You abandon yourself by turning away from who you are as an individual.
- You focus on what others might think or approve of and stop caring for yourself physically and emotionally.
- You do for others before you do for yourself, because you believe others are more important and more deserving.

By rejecting and abandoning yourself, you do to yourself what you are afraid others will eventually do to you. Doing something negative to yourself first doesn't seem to hurt as much.

These two crucial aspects of self-rejection and self-abandonment interfere with maintaining healthy, natural eating patterns. As you learn how to be more accepting of yourself and how to pull your focus inward, you will find that the changes you want to make regarding your eating patterns become easier and more permanent. They will begin to come about because you <u>want</u> them to happen. This occurs when you begin to truly believe that you deserve to have them happen.

Non-natural vs. Natural Eating Patterns

Now that you have a better idea about where your focus has been and what kind of personal environment you have surrounded yourself with, we'll explore eating patterns. If you go to the checklist on Page (ii) of the Appendix and check off all that apply to you, you will recognize how out of touch you have been with your body's food and eating messages. The more statements you checked, the farther away you are from listening to and focusing on what your body tells you is best for it.

Remember the earlier analogy about how a baby eats? This is how <u>you</u> started eating. You let someone know when you were hungry. You ate the foods you wanted and refused the foods you didn't. You spit out the nipple when you were full. You had a definite, natural sense about how much and what kinds of food were enough at any given time.

In your body/brain you have a hunger gauge that gives you the messages about when it's time to fuel up and when it's time to stop. Your stomach feels empty when you are hungry and not empty when you are full, and the rest of your body provides you with feedback about what kinds of food are best for it. Some examples of feedback include an upset stomach from eating too much or the wrong kinds of food, the headache you get after eating too much sugar or waiting too long to eat, or the

"Ahhh -- that really hit the spot" feeling you enjoy after eating just enough of the right kinds of foods for your body.

These feedback messages tell you a lot about what and how much you're putting into your body and what your body thinks of it. If you haven't listened to your stomach and body lately, it may take some practice to hear what they are saying. The difference is eating for natural instead of non-natural reasons.

Awareness of how you have been eating and what a more natural eating pattern looks like is a positive start to making that difference. Without becoming aware of what has been hurting you, you don't know what needs to be changed. Your only alternative is continuing to do what hasn't worked.

Along with becoming aware of what's hurting you, it's important to realize what natural eating actually looks like. Natural eating involves three steps:

1. *Eat when you are hungry.*
2. *Eat what your body needs.*
3. *Stop eating when you are full.*

These three steps are all there is to natural eating. It may seem simple, but putting these steps into practice can be very difficult. They involve being in touch with your body's messages, trusting and respecting those messages, and matching them with appropriate eating behaviors. As you continue this program, you'll learn how to achieve them.

Food = Fuel

The messages you received from others about putting food into your body are a big part of what has kept you trapped in non-natural, self-destructive eating patterns and judgmental belief systems. Messages such as, "Clean your plate," "I made this just for you," and "Children are starving in China," have blocked you from hearing your own body's messages. These old messages have also covered up your body's natural relationship with food. That relationship is very simple and very basic: **Food Equals Fuel.** This statement is not meant to take the enjoyment out of eating, but simply to acknowledge food's originally uncomplicated position regarding your body.

In the past you may have looked at food and eating as a way to please others, rebel against others, take back control, or escape from feelings and situations you are uncomfortable with. Instead of using food as a way to nourish your body, you have used it as a way to try to nurture and protect yourself. You have used food for something it's not made for -- a problem solver. Unfortunately, using food and eating in this manner prevents your real problems from being resolved.

Using food for anything but hunger and nourishment is using food in a self-destructive way. You have subconsciously learned to use food or the rejection of food as an aid for most uncomfortable situations. You've learned to cover up any uncomfortable emotions by eating or not allowing yourself to eat, When you use food to attempt to solve problems or to distract you from emotions and situations you find uncomfortable, you allow the real problem to remain unexplored, hoping it will just go away. It doesn't go away; it keeps triggering more non-natural eating patterns.

Bringing up some of those subconscious beliefs to a conscious level will allow you to take a look at them in a more concrete way. By making them conscious you will be able to grab hold of them more readily in order to confront them and ultimately change them into something more positive. With a more positive belief system on all levels, you will find eating patterns and food choices changing without feeling deprived or forced into doing something you really don't want to do.

The Mirror of Your Mind

So far you have identified where your focus is, what kind of belief system you have been functioning under, and in what kind of personal environment you have been trying to grow and change. You are now aware of what natural eating entails, and just how far away you are from it.

None of this is intended to discourage you. Instead, the more information you have at hand about what is going on with you, the more real it becomes. It's when we keep a lot of what we do and think inside, instead of exposing it to the light, that we have the most difficult time changing. This unwillingness to look at our own reality fosters denial of the extent and depth of the problem.

It's only when you become willing to take a look at the reality of your situation that you will be able to make the changes and adjustments you want. As you become more familiar with your perceptions and attitudes about food and eating, it will be easier for you to pinpoint where your problem areas are. Making these perceptions more real for yourself is one way to become more familiar with and accepting of them.

One perception of yourself includes the image you have of what your body looks like. It's like looking in a mirror in your mind: what do you see when you look in that mirror? An exercise that can help you make the image more real is to draw on paper what you have been "seeing" in your mental mirror.

Often, the image we carry doesn't coincide with the reality of our bodies. We may mentally see ourselves in a better or worse light than we really are. My own mental image was that of a green and orange pear. My body doesn't really look like a pear, but that's how I visualized it. Your mental image can take the shape of a human body perhaps with exaggerated features; an animal; a fruit or vegetable; an abstract *thing*.

In order to get that mental image out of your head and into reality, you must first make it real for yourself. One exercise that can help you accomplish this is to draw a picture of how you see yourself in the mirror of your mind: Draw the mental image of how you look onto Page (iii) of the Appendix. Let yourself go with this exercise. Use colors where they show up in your mind. Don't think about it too much. Just let the image flow through your arm and out your fingers onto the piece of paper. In this way you can actually look at your body image and begin to see how it is affecting your perception of yourself. Do this *before* you continue reading.

Picture Your Body

I don't claim to be able to tell you what your picture means. Only you know what the underlying meaning of your drawing is. If there is something there you don't understand or that disturbs you, you might want to take it to a therapist for help with the interpretation. As an idea, though, here are some insights that have been shared by others when doing this exercise.

What does your picture look like? Is it realistic? Is it judgmental? Is it romanticized? (One woman pictured herself as a "Rubenesque" Venus. She used this as a way to cover up how much she disliked her body size.)

What kinds of colors did you use? Red can mean anger, blue can mean sadness, green can mean growth, yellow can mean fear. Was it stark black and white? No color may mean that you feel you have a colorless existence, or that you don't deserve color. Was your picture in colors you don't really like? Did you emphasize the parts of you that you think are the worst? Several people have shared that this was a clue to how focused they've come to be on the parts of themselves they believe aren't good enough.

Did you draw a person? If so, were any of the body parts left out? A person with no feet can mean a sense of not being grounded, not being solid with yourself. A person without clothes could indicate a more comfortable feeling about one's body.

Not drawing a person at all could indicate one's creative forces at work. It could also mean discomfort with oneself as a person or a feeling of not being able to assert personal boundaries.

These insights are only to be taken as suggestions. You can interpret them as you like or get help with them from a counselor or therapist if you choose. Your mental image and its meaning are totally personal and individual. There is no right or wrong way to see yourself. This is simply a means of gathering information.

The next exercise is designed to get some of your emotions out of your head and onto paper. Drawing them helps you to acknowledge and sort out just what it is you feel about having the body you have. On the Page (iv) of the Appendix, draw your feelings about how you perceive your body. Don't use words at this time, but draw symbols or pictures about how you feel regarding how you look.

Again, just let those emotions emerge from your mind, stream through your arm, and out your fingers onto the page. The less you think about it and the more you just let it flow, the more you will be able to learn about yourself. Do this before you go on reading.

Picture Your Emotions

Once again, notice the colors you used. Acknowledge to yourself the degree of difficulty you had depicting your emotions. One woman drew a box wrapped with a red ribbon. She stated that she tries never to let her feelings out, and therefore has a hard time even knowing which ones are there. This woman eventually talked to a therapist about this aspect of her emotions as it related to her eating problems. What she found was that she was suffering from bulimia, and was then able to get the help she needed.

Different people have used different symbols and colors to represent their feelings. Raindrops and blue were often symbolic of sadness. Red and straight lines represented anger. Squiggly lines and many colors showed confusion. Black tornados or holes indicated shame and hiding. Green showed hope. Yellow could be hope, happiness, or fear. Squares and rectangles often signified a feeling of being trapped or closed in. Disliked colors usually symbolized feelings of unworthiness.

Feelings can be difficult for many people to get in touch with. So many times we have been told not to be sad or angry, so we hide those feelings away as if they were bad or shameful. It's important to remember that feelings are what make us human. Honoring all our feelings gives us a sense of empathy and compassion for others as well as for ourselves.

The third exercise is one that works with words. On Page (v) of the Appendix, write down the words you would use to describe your body. Don't attempt to edit these words. Just let them emerge from your mind and onto the paper. Do this exercise before you continue reading.

Describe Your Body

Look at how negative and judgmental these words are. The concept of putting personally negative judgments on your body gives you an idea of the perceptions you have learned to associate with something that is not perfect. The more negatively judgmental these words are, the more difficult it is for you to care about and for yourself.

These three exercises give you a more reality-based idea of the personal environment you have surrounded yourself with. Bringing these beliefs into reality by getting them out of your head and onto paper enables you to see them as they are. This awareness of exactly what has been going on with you allows you to decide if you want to make changes, and if so, what kinds of changes.

The choice is up to you. There's nothing bad or good about your decision. Knowing what you've been up against, however, allows you the reality of where you are now. In turn, you have a more solid base from which to make your decision. It's okay if you're not ready at this time. What's important is that you go at your own pace. After all, this is your individual process.

Don't worry if you weren't able to do any of these exercises, either. Learning about ourselves can be scary, difficult, and/or confusing. You may not be ready for that yet, and that's ok. Each and every one of us has their own history, triggers, and beliefs. Some will find this more difficult to do than others, while some may find it impossible to do at this time.

There is nothing wrong with you if you're not ready to do any of this yet. You may have issues that keep you from digging too deeply. When you're ready is the time for you to do what you want about any of this. There is no shame or blame here. Do what you can when you are ready and able.

Change takes not only the courage to look at your reality, but also the willingness to risk doing something different from the familiar. A decision to change means that at this point in your life you are ready and able to do what's necessary to leave old attitudes and behaviors behind. A decision not to change means that at this point in your life you are just not ready or able, no matter the reason. Knowing your limitations is just as important as knowing your strengths.

If you have decided to begin making changes at this time, read on. This program is focused on change. Knowing what has been holding you back from change is what you have learned from the previous exercises and checklists. The assignments for this lesson are directed toward lessening those beliefs and attitudes that have kept you trapped in the destructive cycle of non-acceptance and negative judgments.

The Start of Something New

Think of the bodies you see when you go to the mall. Many of these bodies are not perfect. However, we usually compare our own body to a body that lives up to an artificial standard of perfection and then berate ourselves for not measuring up to that standard. Is the attainment of perfection the only time you believe you deserve to be kind to yourself?

You can abuse yourself mentally (your drawing of your body), emotionally (your drawing of your feelings) and verbally (your list of words). Will you only care for and about your body when it is perfect? When is that? A certain size? A specific weight? A particular shape?

The fact is, your body changes all through your life. It doesn't look the same now as it did when you were 7 years old and it won't look the same now as it will when you are 87. Surgery, illness, and accidents can all change the shape of your body and its parts. And even if everyone weighed the same, we'd all still be different sizes and shapes.

Being able to look at your body today, knowing that it is worth care and love, may be one of the hardest tasks you will attempt throughout the course of this program. That is why the issue of acceptance must be addressed from the beginning.

Think of your best friend. Do you accept their body as just being a part of who they are? Do you see them as being a good person even with an imperfect body? Most of us accept our friend's body as simply their body, without it being a judgment of them as a person. You deserve no less. You deserve to care about your body no matter what it looks like. Your body deserves care and kindness no matter what shape it has.

This is the basis of acceptance. To accept your body as is permits you to care for and about your body, whatever shape or size it happens to be at this moment. Acceptance allows you to acknowledge that even with imperfections, your body is worth your love. And it is through love that change is encouraged to take place.

So it is through acceptance that the first step toward change happens. Have you been able to change by keeping a non-accepting personal environment around yourself? Has change happened when you demean yourself, ignore yourself, or put yourself down for not being perfect? Maybe it's time to modify your approach.

Creating a non-judgmental, caring personal environment takes time and courage. It's risky to begin allowing acceptance of something you've been taught to reject and abandon. It's scary to turn toward the very thing you've been trained to turn away from.

Your First Assignment

The first assignment may not be easy. If you have read this far, however, you have all that it takes to begin. If you are ready to tackle something new and different regarding your food, eating, and body image, you're at the right place.

The first assignment starts you on the road to acceptance. Acceptance is a process and therefore won't be realized overnight. It may never happen completely. Your goal is to eventually be consistently accepting of your body as it is in the moment. We are looking for progress, not perfection. Some days it just won't happen, but you can reach a point where it will happen far more often than not.

- Get a full-length mirror for your house if you don't have one. Many people with body image issues don't keep a mirror available because they don't want to see all of themselves at one time, while others, if they do have one, keep it in order to harshly judge and criticize themselves.
- Look at yourself in the mirror from top to bottom on a daily basis and say the words "I accept my body." <u>Use just those four words.</u>

Having your clothes on or off or saying the words aloud or in your head are both your call. The important thing is to begin the process of acceptance without judgment.

Acceptance means allowing yourself to care about your body no matter what its physical appearance. Just as you care about your friends and treat them with kindness and concern no matter what the size or shape of their bodies, you deserve no less.

To Remember

- Change means risk. To risk is to take a step into the unknown. Stepping into the unknown allows you to widen your "corridor of happiness"
- The narrower your "corridor of happiness," the more miserable you will remain
- Natural eating consists of three steps:
  1. *Eat when you're hungry*
  2. *Eat what your body needs*
  3. *Stop eating when you're full*
- Your body will tell you everything you need to know about nourishing it
- Comparisons are used only to make you feel better or worse than someone else. If your self-esteem is where it belongs, you don't need to compare
- Judgments encourage you to remain surrounded by a negative personal environment, shutting out the reality of all that's true and positive about you
- Acceptance means caring for and about yourself even while you're not perfect

CHAPTER II

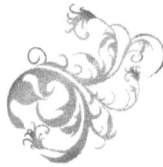

THE DIET DECISION

Assignment Review

People have reported varying degrees of difficulty with this first assignment from Chapter I. For some, it was impossible. For others, there was very little problem. Some stopped after a day or two; others were able to continue throughout the week. For everyone, I encourage continuation with this assignment. This is the beginning of change on many levels.

If you have been taught not to be happy or satisfied unless you achieve perfection, you may have also been taught to reject or abandon anything that is less than perfect, or to continue working at it until it becomes perfect. Imperfections may be viewed as sins, failures, or personal weaknesses. Accepting someone or something as good enough and working with what you have "as is" may feel unacceptable.

If the idea that you are and always will be imperfect by virtue of being human means you are not allowed to accept yourself the way you are, you will continue to be pretty miserable throughout your life. It's only by learning how to accept that being human means you will never be perfect, and there's nothing wrong with that which allows you to care about all the parts of you.

Acceptance doesn't mean things can't or won't change. Acceptance doesn't denote resignation or defeat. What acceptance does is allow you to care for and care about something even though it isn't perfect. It's an acknowledgment that while perfection can't be attained, improvements can certainly be ongoing. However, because improvements are positive, they will rarely flourish in a negative environment.

Turning a pattern of negativity and non-acceptance around takes time and energy. You're working against years of practice and beliefs. Like anything new, acceptance becomes more comfortable with time. The goal you are trying to reach is acceptance of your body as a naturally flawed yet wonderful organism, one that deserves care no matter what it looks like.

Acceptance is a recognition of reality that leaves room for change. Acceptance allows you to continue caring about and for your body no matter what shape it's in. Even if we all weighed the same, our bodies would look different from each other's. By accepting your body, you begin to eliminate judgments and negativity and help provide a gentle, kind, and caring environment in which to live, work, grow, and change.

Some people *seem* to have no problem saying accepting words to themselves. They usually explain this by saying that they've adopted a "the hell with you" attitude and decided they were going to be OK with their bodies in spite of what anyone else says.

Be careful about this type of attitude. It may simply be one of denial. On the surface it sounds like no one's approval is needed. Inside, however, that approval from others is still wanted very much. This type of thinking is used as a protective wall against the pain of not getting outside approval. While it may look good on the outside, it doesn't ring true *inside*. For acceptance to have real meaning, it must come from inside yourself with no denial, defenses, or negative attitudes.

Acceptance also acknowledges that change will happen to your body which is outside your control. It allows you to remain comfortable with your body even while it goes through natural or unavoidable changes during your life. Your body changes on a day-to-day basis. The more accepting you are of this fact, the more comfortable you will be with its imperfections along the way. Here are some examples of how change in your life can change your body:

➢ **Age** -- your body looks and functions one way at 7 years old and differently at 37 or at 87. Changes within internal functions, such as cell reproduction and repair rates, will cause changes in external appearance.

➢ **Outside intervention** –sun damage or other environmental factors, surgery, medications, and accidents can drastically change both your body's ability to function as well as its physical appearance.

➢ **Natural functions** -- hormone fluctuations, menstrual cycles, pregnancy, childbirth, metabolism rates, stress, and illnesses all affect how your body looks and operates.

➢ **Behavior choices** -- eating patterns, as well as amounts and types of exercise, change your body's shape and appearance.

Even while it changes, your body deserves the care that comes with acceptance. After all it is the human body you have been entrusted with to care for and nurture in this lifetime. Your body doesn't deserve to be abandoned or rejected simply because it doesn't look "perfect."

One way to look at acceptance is to compare caring about your body to caring about children. If you accept that children are individuals, each with their own unique talents and quirks, you can also accept that children are individuals who happen to come in all shapes and sizes. There isn't any blueprint for the "right" or "perfect" child.

These "imperfect" children can be loved, cared about, and cared for. They need encouragement to grow and change with respect for their differences and imperfections. Child rearing books continually suggest that gentleness and patience, as well as an approach that positively acknowledges skills and talents, be emphasized when the goal is personal improvement and increased self-esteem.

Creating a positive environment for children in which to grow and change aids the process along. Negativity impedes it. It's the acceptance of differences and imperfections that encourages a positive environment, thereby encouraging positive personal growth and change.

If you haven't been able to change your eating habits while being negatively focused on and judgmental to yourself, maybe negative is no longer the way to go. You may want to try something different. Accepting your body as is, and caring for it regardless of its size or shape is the first step to breaking your old, destructive cycle.

Having others in your life who are also non-judgmental about your body is a way to reinforce your own newly accepting messages. Surrounding yourself with encouraging, supportive people and keeping exposure to those who repeat judgmental, negative messages to a minimum will increase your chances of reaching body acceptance more quickly.

Acceptance will not happen overnight. Acceptance is a process. You will not be perfect at it, but the sooner you start and the more you practice, the easier it will get and the faster it will happen. This is where you begin to take control of your eating. You are the determining factor in what you believe from now on.

Tuning In – Changing Your Focus

As you start accepting your body as a living, changing organism instead of a freak to be rejected and abandoned, you open the door to hearing all the information your body gives you about how it is feeling-- cold, hot, comfortable, tired, sore, hungry, full, etc. This information, in turn, is what you are able to use to care for your body in the ways it needs and deserves care. This is the beginning of trust in and respect for your body as unique and individual.

Listening to your body's messages about food and eating tells you not only **when** your body is hungry or full, but also **what** it is hungry for. The more you listen to your body's messages, the easier it is to focus on what your own individual needs are. The more you focus on what your body says, the less you will do what is unhealthy for it.

As you focus on yourself and what your body tells you, you will notice that you begin making more choices that are determined naturally by your body. These choices include food amounts and types your body tells you are healthiest for it. However, you need to be cautious when listening to body messages. Often your mouth or eyes will give you messages about food *they* want. When this happens and you feed your body for reasons other than physical hunger, you are probably eating in a non-natural way. There is most likely an underlying issue that you are trying to distract yourself from or bury.

Think about animals in the wild. While they are surrounded by food, they pick and choose which and how much they will eat. Their bodies, in order to maintain the weight that's best for them, tell them when they are hungry, what they are hungry for, and how much is sufficient. It's all built into their natural regulatory system.

Being animals as well, it's the same for us. If we listen, our bodies will tell us all we need to know concerning food and eating. It all depends where your focus is. When you focus outside yourself for messages about when, what, and how much to eat, you will end up eating in a non-natural manner and your body will reflect that in some way, shape, or form. You have the choice to either continue focusing outside yourself, worrying about messages and standards set forth by others, or to begin pulling that focus into yourself and your body.

How Did the Focus Get Away From You in the First Place?

Some of those outside messages and standards are shown to you every day through media images. Those pictures show you that losing weight is the key to being attractive, lovable, and happy. Models and other celebrities invariably look slim, trim, and in great physical shape. The message is that these types of shapes are the keys to your own sense of happiness and success.

The problem is that these are all images being projected for your viewing pleasure, and images aren't reality. Airbrushing, special lighting, makeup and wardrobe experts, as well as surgical procedures, are all utilized to make these images look perfect. These people are paid to look happy and healthy. On Page (vi) of the Appendix is an excerpt from a 2019 interview with Douglas Rushkoff, author of *Team Human*. He talks about how technology, going back to TV, and advertising has endeavored to keep us unhappy with ourselves, thereby buying into images and messages of unattainable perfection.

Unhealthy eating patterns and lifestyles, cigarettes, and drugs are all ways that famous people have admitted to in order to project such images. Personal trainers, dietitians, and in-home gyms are utilized and paid for, and schedules are rearranged in order to accommodate their regular use. For these people, having a perfect image is part of the job.

Image is not necessarily substance, however. Physical health and emotional well-being are not dependent on images. Instead, they depend on messages your body sends you regarding how you feel in any given situation.

Physical health and emotional well-being depend on insight and bodily messages, while physical image depends on outside messages and comparisons. If you are taught from very young not to listen to and trust the messages your body gives you, you will learn to listen to and believe the messages that others give you. These "others" include the media advertising messages, which reinforce the lessons you've learned at a very young age about disregarding what your body says.

Here are some examples of how the messages heard as children can influence perceptions and beliefs about food and eating and encourage a continuation of looking outside yourself for the answers you seek:

- I heard a story about a mom telling her nine-month old son who didn't want to eat his peas that he should eat them and appreciate them because there are so many starving children in the world. This mom was using guilt to teach her son to look outside himself for a reason to eat something he not only didn't like, but also that he may have been too full to want.

- A similar situation involved a little girl and her dad. She asked him for something to eat. He told her she wasn't hungry. She said she was; he told her she couldn't be because she had just eaten breakfast. She said she hadn't eaten very much; he told her that she had eaten cereal and toast. She insisted she hadn't eaten very much of either; he told her to wait till later. This dad was teaching his daughter to believe *his* messages about her hunger rather than her own.

- Many people have been told that if they clean their plate they will be "good" boys and girls, or that wasting food is a sin. Equating eating with personal worth or a vision of one's personal eternity gives a person strong motivation for ignoring their own body's messages out of fear.

- How many family reunions encourage people to eat out of a sense of being able to control someone else's emotions? The idea of having a second helping or eating a certain dish that "mom slaved over a hot stove all day to make" sends a message of power. It tells you that you have the power to change another person's emotions just by eating. No wonder so many of us believe we are able to control the uncontrollable.

These kinds of messages helped to shape our perception of the purpose of food and eating in our lives. We learned to attribute all kinds of non-natural functions to what and how we ate. We came to believe that we can change someone's emotions or life experience through our food consumption, that we cannot rely on and trust our own body's messages, and that the way we want to eat isn't good enough. We ended up believing that we are bad or good people because of what and how much we eat.

Although many people like to blame the media for causing unnatural body shapes and sizes as something to strive for in order to be happy, I believe the messages about striving for happiness by focusing outside yourself began at a very young age. When you get messages that teach you to deny what your body is saying to you, to look outside yourself for reasons to eat or not, and that encourage you to strive for approval from others early on, you learn to believe that others know what is best for you.

This sets you up to believe that media messages are the ones to believe, not the messages that come from inside you. Media messages don't have any power if you don't believe them. They don't have any power if you acknowledge that their job is to sell products and fantasy.

When you are invested in reality, you know that the only messages that make true sense for you in the long run are those that come from within. This is not to say that fantasy doesn't have its place. It's refusing to acknowledge fantasy as fantasy, enjoying it for a bit, but returning to and living in reality that can become problematic. Living in reality allows you to make decisions and choices that will truly enhance your life and promote well-being and happiness from within.

Diets for Physical Health and Physical Image

The reality of diets is that they are essentially of two types -- those that are concerned with numbers (Physical Image Diets or PIDs) and those that are concerned with the individual needs of your body (Physical

Health Diets or PHDs). There is a big difference between the two.

For one thing, numbers-based diets are used to maintain an image. They are mainly concerned with the "right" size and weight of a body and are dictated by numbers. Many ads for physical image diets also give you the impression that once you reach this "right" size or weight, you will be happy because other people will want to be in your life. You will find true love, make the best business deals, or just generally enjoy yourself with others looking at you appreciatively. You begin to believe that once your body is approved of by others, you will find and express the "you" that has been hidden for so long.

PIDs are also almost totally focused on numbers: weight, calories, pounds gained and lost, clothing size, etc. With the focus on numbers, you disregard any messages your body sends you if it contradicts the numerical goal you have set your sights on. This is how you are kept out of touch with your body and its messages and forced to focus outside yourself. Once again you're being taught to abandon your body and what it's telling you.

This is not to say PIDs aren't good for anything. They are extremely good at helping you lose weight because their rules and restrictions are focused on weight loss. If losing weight is your primary goal, a physical image diet is what you want.

After losing weight, however, many people realize that they have not achieved the happiness and well-being these diets have promised. They're still afraid of conflict, they still fear being alone, and they are still un-comfortable with emotional intimacy in relationships. To cope with these fears and discomforts, they often return to the choices and behaviors that helped them through uncomfortable situations in the past -- non-natural eating patterns and food choices. This is why they regain all the weight they've just lost.

Diets that focus on physical image are also good for allowing you to look like you're doing something about your weight problem. Whenever you say you're on a diet, you are giving people the message they don't have to tell you that you need to do something about your weight -- you're already doing it.

What you *don't* get from physical image diets are happiness, love, or a lot of good friends -- these things can only come from you. They come from how you feel about yourself and your life, and how you present yourself to others. If you believe a certain body shape is what will make you happy, you will feel miserable and negative toward yourself anytime you don't have that body shape. When you feel miserable about yourself, you will present yourself less confidently, less personably, and more restrictively. You will also eat in a non-natural way once again.

If you want to learn how to eat differently for your life, it may be time to try something different. This is where a diet focused on your physical health comes in. A physical health diet is determined by the internal needs of your body. It is basically the opposite dynamic of the physical image diet. When you eat for your health and well-being, your body determines the diet instead of the diet determining your body. Diets that are concerned with your physical health are not concerned with a "right" size or weight. Your size and weight adjust themselves by what's best for your body.

PHDs enhance your physical health by maintaining the focus on your body and what is best for it. Any restrictions are those that are dictated by your body. An example is the diabetic's diet. Sugar is eliminated from the diabetic's diet because their body doesn't do well with it, not because of an image diet's dictation. Another example is someone who has problems with high blood pressure; this body is also saying that eating certain foods is dangerous. It's not the diet that is telling the body what it needs but the other way around.

In both cases, the battle for control is won by personal choice. A person eliminates what is unhealthy because they care about themselves, instead of because it's what's expected. When you eliminate by choice, you regain and maintain control of what you eat. You are not controlled by the diet; instead, you are the one who is actually in control. We give up trying to control the effects of the food through its elimination rather than by trying to control its intake.

The difference between a numbers-based and a body message-based diet is critical. A diet used to maintain an image continues the training that was started long ago -- that you shouldn't trust yourself, you can't control your eating, you're weak, something's wrong with you, or that you're just not good enough the way you are. It teaches you to get a body shape based on societal rather than health standards. It maintains the lose/gain cycle by reinforcing your mistrust in your body and its messages. You are only allowed to feel good about yourself when the scale gives you permission or when your numerical goal is reached. This diet is concerned with weight loss and numbers, which makes health and well-being secondary.

A diet to maintain physical health, however, is essential to your survival and well-being. It heeds your body's messages about restrictions based on what does or doesn't agree with your body, and is based on self-respect. Ignoring these messages is self-destructive and can be life-threatening. You feel good about yourself because you are taking care of yourself, not because you look a certain way. This diet is concerned with your health and well-being, and numbers are secondary. This diet is for your life.

Eating for physical health is a gift you give yourself -- a gift of respect and caring. When it comes to true personal happiness, caring for and about yourself is the foundation upon which such happiness is built.

Food as Reward and Punishment

As you have seen, image diets have personal judgments attached to them. These diets seem to tell you that when you get down to a certain size or lose a certain number of pounds you have been "good," while if you gain weight or go beyond that size you have been "bad."

Many of us have been taught to believe we deserve to be punished when we do something "bad." Going to bed without eating or having our favorite foods withheld ("You don't get any ice cream because you pulled your sister's hair.") have been punishments that deprived us of favorite foods when someone decided we were "naughty." We often use food deprivation as the means of self-punishment in the same way.

Withholding food from yourself as punishment paves the way for out-of-control eating. If food restrictions are viewed as *punishment* for being "bad," then letting loose of all restrictions when it comes to food or eating can be viewed as a *reward* for being "good." As soon as we put food and eating into a reward and punishment category, we immediately take the focus off our bodies and their needs. We stop looking at food as a source of nourishment.

Often it is the numbers on the scale that determine if you've been "bad" or "good." The punishment ends when the scale says so. When you hit the right number, you can reward yourself for all your willpower by eating all the food you have been denied. Instead of focusing on how your body feels and what it needs, your focus has been on what you haven't been allowed to eat and on how deprived you've been all the while you've been on that diet.

Being focused on rewarding yourself for your dietary accomplishments leads to the same patterns of eating as before. You give yourself permission to eat what your mouth wants instead of what your body needs. If you are like the vast majority of people who lose weight on a numbers-based diet, you will eventually regain all the weight you lost, and more. Of course, when this happens, you feel "bad" once again and it's time for another punishment. The lose/gain cycle has perpetuated itself under the guise of childhood patterns of rewards and punishment for good/bad behavior.

This cycle returns once your goal weight is reached and the diet has ended because you have no other choice but to return to your original eating habits and patterns. Neither your perception of what to eat nor why to eat have changed. Your focus remains on food and eating rather than on your body and its needs. Only the numbers have changed.

Taking Control

Believing you must pay for your sins is the basis for the lose-gain cycle you're so familiar with. Giving your weight the authority to determine your "goodness" and "badness" as a person keeps you feeling that you have no power of choice for yourself. You become resigned to being either at one extreme of the diet cycle or the other. You are either in control when you're on a diet, or you're out of control when you're not. There is no in-between. You turn to an image diet to take control for you because you don't believe you have the willpower or the strength to control your eating yourself.

When you follow an image diet, you are saying in effect, "O Great Diet, tell me what to do. You must know better than I what is good for me and my body." Unfortunately, the opposite is true. The image diet *doesn't* know. *You* are the only one who can hear your body's messages. A numbers-based diet is not designed to change your regular eating patterns, belief systems, or perceptions about what food and eating mean to you. Without these changes, however, you return to the only eating patterns you know once the diet is over.

Staying Stuck

Why not break the cycle? Why, if it doesn't work for you, do you keep doing the same thing over and over? Seems kind of strange when you stop and think about it, doesn't it? Yet that is what millions of people around the world are doing at any given moment.

One factor that plays a part in keeping you stuck in the cycle may involve a fear of change. You continue playing into an unspoken go-nowhere dynamic -- *if it doesn't work, do more of it.* Although your experiences with diets have been negative, you've attained some degree of comfort with them. At least you know what to expect!

This procedure is connected to a comfort factor that you may be trying to maintain. Even if image diets don't work for you, they are familiar. They feel safer and more comfortable than doing something different. You might not like them, but diets based on numbers are what you know how to deal with. They tell you what to do or not to do, and you're used to that. After all, it's something you've been doing most all your life.

Another factor that may keep you in the destructive cycle is the idea of belonging. As soon as you begin a diet, you can feel like you "belong," that you are part of a community of suffering and cheating. Anywhere you go, you will meet people who speak your language--"Oh, I really shouldn't."; "I can't--I'm on a diet."; "Maybe I'll have just one. One won't hurt." Dieting gives you an instant bond to another dieter.

A third factor involves the concept of getting "in shape." Many people talk about getting in shape instead of dieting. Low-fat/no-fat foods and exercise are being used as ways to lose weight instead of the idea that a nutritionally-balanced diet and moderate exercise are essential for maintaining a healthy body.

A final factor involves our love affair with the "quick fix." We want our "cure" for unhappiness to be easy and fast. We want to believe that simply by losing weight we will find the happiness and love that has been eluding us. After all, the ads *say* image diets are the answer, the pictures *look* like they're the answer, and the people who give the testimonials make us want to *believe* they're the answer.

But our own experience has told us that image diets <u>don't</u> make us happy. They help us lose weight, but that's all. What they don't do is show us how to eat in a way that is self-respectful. Unfortunately, because we have been taught to rely on diets for a sense of "being in control," we are left with the belief that we only have two options:

1) DIET!
2) BE OUT OF CONTROL!

Therein lies your dilemma. This is why you keep going back to dieting again and again, remaining stuck in that lose/gain cycle. You believe it is you who are the failure instead of the diets.

Breaking the Cycle

To extricate yourself from this dilemma requires risk and change. Change can be scary and it is stressful. Change means saying good-bye to something known and comfortable and saying hello to something new and different. Changing self-destructive eating patterns and food choices means taking a realistic look at those messages that have ruled your food and eating habits. It means eliminating those messages that don't work for you anymore and creating your own. It means taking back true control.

The first step, then, in breaking the lose/gain cycle is to become aware of the kinds of messages that have helped to keep you trapped. You have been holding on to messages that have been dictating food, eating, and body image policies to you for many years. These messages cause you to go against your body's messages, and you end up hurting yourself both physically and emotionally.

These messages have usually come from other people, often out of care and concern for your health and well-being ("Clean your plate before you have dessert"), or out of care and concern for someone else's feelings ("Aunt Martha will be so hurt if you don't at least have one piece of her pie"). As an adult now, it's up to you to determine how much you want to take care of yourself physically, what taking care of yourself physically actually means, and how you actually want to show care and concern for others' feelings. *You* are the one with the final choice as to what you do or do not put into your mouth. *You* can decide if eating what you're not hungry for is the way to show someone you love them. In the end, your body is *your* responsibility, not anyone else's.

If you accept that some of your old messages about body image, food, and eating aren't beneficial for your health and well-being, then you may be ready to take control. You are the only one who is able to break the lose/gain cycle, and to regain the power others' messages have held over you.

The Power of Old Messages

The real power of these messages lies within the realm of your mind, the perception you have of what they mean to you as an individual. Many of the messages you have received throughout your life represent some form of control and authority. In order to be loved and accepted by those who had authority over you, you believed it was necessary to adhere to their rules and do what they told you.

Our need to be accepted and loved by others is a basic necessity of human beings. We need to feel we belong. Belonging to a group (whether it's family of origin, family of choice, among friends, at the office, part of a couple, etc. – it doesn't matter) gives us a sense of feeling seen and acknowledged.

When relating this to the power of old messages about food and eating, we have tried to eat in the ways these messages have told us to in order to feel that we belong. When we feel that people won't reject or abandon us because we are doing what they want, we believe that we are then OK. This is powerful indeed!

Rejection and abandonment are two demons in life that people constantly struggle to escape because they cause pain. This pain is something we would rather inflict on ourselves through self-rejection and self-abandonment because we know how to deal with self-inflicted pain much easier than the pain of someone else inflicting it on us. We would much rather eat the way someone else wants us to eat, (whether it's by way of messages from parents, teachers, friends, society, or the media) even though it doesn't feel good to us. At least we know they won't reject or abandon us if we do what they want.

This may sound contradictory, especially in light of the fact that many of those messages tell us to lose weight, don't eat so much, or that we're too skinny. This is where your individuality comes in. You as an individual take the messages that are the most authoritative to you and follow them to the letter. The messages that if you don't follow them will have the direst consequences for you and your life are the ones with the most authority and control over you. These are the messages that have the power.

These messages will not necessarily be the same for everyone. For some, messages about cleaning your plate are the strongest. For others, messages about how bad it is to be fat will have the most power. Some people believe wasting food by throwing the excess away is a sin. Others believe that remaining a certain size or weight is what will bring them love and happiness.

The fears attached to such messages and many more like them are what have the ultimate control over you. You will need to examine your own messages in order to discover what it is you fear. In the above examples, it may be that you are afraid to lose the relationship with your mother if you don't eat the way she taught you (you are continuing to be the good child she always wanted). You may be afraid others will look at you with disgust if you become fat (you may have seen someone you care about do this). Your religious background may deem sinners to endless suffering (better to suffer now than for all eternity). You may be afraid that you will end up alone (who wants someone that isn't as desirable as all the models and stars on TV?)

The power of these and many other messages can be overwhelming. They go to the heart of your being and insecurities. It is when you begin to explore these messages in a realistic way, examining them for their specific meaning to you as an individual, that you begin to stimulate your own sense of power.

Reclaiming Your Personal Power

The assignment for this chapter is twofold, and is designed to enable you to begin reclaiming your own sense of personal power. First, it's important to grab hold of those old messages in order to look them square in the eye and realize what you've been up against. To do this, make a list of all the messages you can think of that have to do with food, eating, or your body that you've heard throughout your life. It is important to write them down in order to put them into a more concrete perspective for yourself.

Be sure to include any messages that have numbers in them (such as good or bad sizes, goal weights, or times to eat or not to eat), should's or shouldn't's (you should always eat a complete breakfast, you shouldn't waste food) and examples your parents may have set for you around food, eating or body image either by word or behavior (did mom diet a lot? Did dad comment on girls' bodies? Did they use food as rewards or take food away as punishments?).

Also include messages that contain the implication of good and bad (chocolate is bad, lettuce is good), definitions (what is a meal? What does going out to eat mean? How does food play a part in social gatherings?), and anything you've ever heard about fat and thin. Include foods used as rewards, expectations about eating, and the meanings you discover behind some of your eating patterns and food choices, especially if they're connected to acceptance and lovability.

Make this list as complete as possible. Use friends as a resource to find out about messages they might remember that you can relate to. Sisters and brothers may be of help with this. Be as thorough as you can. The more complete this list is now, the more completely you will be able to release yourself from these messages later. A guide to help you include as many messages as possible is on Page (vii) of the Appendix.

Once this list is as complete as you can make it, move on to Chapter III. Ideally, it is best to take a week for this assignment before going on to the next chapter in order for you to notice how the information in this chapter plays out in your life on a day-to-day basis. This time also allows you to process what you have learned and put into practice whatever fits for you before going on to the next chapter and new information.

The second part of the assignment for this week is an action assignment. If you have used your scale as a determining factor in feeling good or bad about yourself, you are using it as a means of acceptance and lovability. If this is the case, put your scale somewhere difficult for you to reach, or give it to someone else for a while. It's important for you to learn to live without those numbers. Giving such authority to the scale keeps you from feeling your own power.

If you want to feel your own power as an adult, remove that so-called authority figure from your life. You don't need anything telling you whether you're good or bad as a person. You are changing your focus to what's best for your health and well-being. Your body will let you know if it's feeling good or not.

Check in with yourself during the week for any emotions or thoughts that come up for you around these assignments. You may want to begin a journal if you haven't already done so. Use your journal as a way of getting to know yourself better. By learning who you are, you become acquainted with your individual strengths and weaknesses. Doing so enables you to regain your sense of self-trust and allows you to begin feeling your sense of personal power. Your power lies in your individuality.

To Remember

- Acceptance is **_not_** resignation
- A diet based on image satisfies the numbers; a diet based on your body's needs satisfies your being
- Food is not a punishment or a reward
- Messages from others about weight and body size have trained you to focus outside yourself
- A fear of change will keep you stuck in your unhealthy ways
- When you follow your body's messages, you regain control of your eating
- Old messages about food and eating have kept you stuck in a self-destructive cycle
- Happy adults consistently do what's best for them
- You have two choices when you eat -- You can either hurt yourself or nourish yourself with food

CHAPTER III

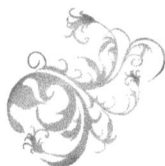

OUT WITH THE OLD, IN WITH THE NEW

Assignment Review

Old Messages

If you followed the assignment suggestion at the end of Chapter II, you now have a list of old messages about food, eating, and body image. It's important to have as many of them written down as possible because this chapter contains an exercise for you to do to help you reduce their power over you.

Besides the types of old messages already mentioned in Chapter II, here are a few categories of messages to be sure to cover:

- Any messages concerning labels that have been put on certain foods, such as "snack" foods, "appetizers," "breakfast" foods, etc. Food is food and *you* get to determine how much and what kind to eat and when. Eat food because of your body's messages, not because of a label attached to it.

- Labels can set up automatic messages to you about how to perceive certain foods which will generate automatic responses from you. These responses cause you to eat according to a preconceived mind-set about the food. For example, how many times have you been full after eating the "appetizer" but you continued to eat because it wasn't the "main meal?"

- Any messages that have to do with guilt or other people's emotions and lives. Eating to make another person happy or from the fear of hurting another person's feelings has nothing to do with your body and its needs. Any time you feel obligated to eat in order to please someone else or so that you won't offend them, you are eating from your head or your heart instead of from your stomach.

- Any messages that include definitions and habits about foods, meals, and eating. Often, they have kept you trapped in a specific perception and behavior that doesn't fit with your body's needs. Take the definition of a meal, for example. Does "meal" always mean a full-course dinner to you? The problem with this is that if you're only hungry for a banana, you may feel unsatisfied mentally because a banana doesn't fit your definition of a meal. That unsatisfied feeling may compel you to eat more than what you're truly hungry for.

- Habits to include on your list involve any rituals or patterns, such as eating in front of the TV or with something to read. They also include situations in which you've given yourself automatic permission to eat in a self-destructive way, such as when socializing, at family get-togethers, after work, late at night, holidays, celebrations, etc.

T-N-T

It's time to take a final look at your list. These messages have encouraged you to be out of touch with your body and its own individual messages. This list gives you an idea about why you haven't known how to eat in a natural, life-enhancing manner. These messages have been your constant companions, and you've had a lot of practice eating according to them.

If these old messages have worked for you, then by all means keep them. You may have been raised by outside rules and regulations all your life, and they feel familiar and comfortable. Having the power to make your own rules can feel very frightening because it's unknown. Feeling empowered may be something you have not had a lot of practice with.

The thought of getting rid of the only messages that you have known concerning food and eating may bring up different emotions for you. You may feel fear, believing these outside controls have been the only things that have kept you from eating and eating until you blew up and exploded. You may feel cynical, believing it's going to take more than a silly exercise to actually get rid of these messages and reduce their power over you. You may feel a sense of relief that at last, something can be done about all this.

Your anxiety may be due to a lack of practice in trusting yourself and your own messages. Can you remember a time when you weren't hungry but everyone else was? You knew it; it was real; but it wasn't the way others felt. Because the others felt differently, however, you may have covered up what you knew to be true, doubted yourself, minimized your own feelings, or even put yourself down. Rarely did you speak up for yourself and not eat.

Messages from your body about hunger are individual and personal, yet they are as valid as anyone else's messages. Your personal messages don't necessarily run on the same schedule as anyone else's so you won't necessarily feel hungry for the same kind of food at the same time as other people. This doesn't make you in any way wrong or strange--it simply emphasizes your individuality.

To tap into your own individuality, however, it is important to remove the messages that came from other people. One way that many have found helpful is by doing the T-N-T exercise—Tear-'N'-Toss. It's an exercise to help remove other people's messages which have kept you trapped in non-natural eating patterns so you are freer to listen to and respect your own body's messages.

If you are ready now to regain the power that is rightfully yours and to free yourself from the messages that have kept you imprisoned, then it's time for T-N-T. Take that list of old messages you wrote down and tear it up into little pieces. Feel the power as you destroy them. These have been big blocks in your life and it takes power to get rid of them. Next, get a container, toss all those little pieces in there, and say good-by to them. Finally, walk them right out of the room, (or have someone do it for you) outside to the trash/recycling, and out of your life.

For anyone concerned about the negativity of these old messages being released by being recycled, it's important to note that once you tear the messages up, you are nullifying their power. What's left is nothing more than paper and ink, which can hurt nothing and no one.

After you complete this exercise, note how you feel. Is there a sense of power? A sense of exhilaration? A sense of feeling lighter? A sense of cynicism or disbelief? A sense of emptiness, confusion, or fear? Any of these emotions may surface. When I did this exercise myself, I remember my hand shaking as I tore those messages up. I felt a sense of emptiness, like there was now a big hole where those messages had been, and I felt scared about what to do next. After all, my entire way of eating was now in that wastebasket.

When you let go of one way of doing things, it's important to fill the emptiness with something else. Whether that "something else" is healthy or unhealthy is up to you. If you don't make a conscious choice to fill that hole with something healthy, it will probably become filled with something self-destructive. In fact, that's what substituting addictions and unhealthy behaviors is all about.

For example, when people quit smoking, they often overeat to fill the hole left by the absence of their cigarettes. Many people who give up life-threatening eating patterns fill the hole with unhealthy exercise practices. People often make these types of unhealthy substitutions because they don't know how to fill the hole with something healthy.

One way to fill the hole left behind by those old messages you have just eliminated is to replace them with healthy messages. Listed here is a list of healthier, more personal messages about yourself and your eating patterns that can take the place of the old, unhealthy messages you no longer have:

1) I eat when I'm hungry.

I eat to fuel my body. I stay in touch with my stomach's messages and wait until I'm hungry before I eat. Eating for any other reason besides hunger is self-destructive. I refuse to hurt myself with food any more.

2) I eat what my body is hungry for.

I try to match my body's needs as closely as possible by checking in with my stomach in order to discover what food will "fit" in it. I deserve to eat only foods that are healthy for my body. I don't confuse thirst with hunger.

3) I stop eating when I'm full.

I stay focused on my stomach's messages instead of the amount of food on my plate. I waste food when I put more food into my stomach than it needs. To eat more than comfortably fits in my stomach is painful. I deserve only a pleasantly full feeling as part of a healthy eating pattern.

4) I acknowledge my fears, assess the situation, and act appropriately.

I assess a situation to determine if there is true danger, in which case it's important to take quick action, or if I am merely feeling uncomfortable, in which case I look for the source of my discomfort in order to stay in reality. Discomfort won't hurt me; danger can. Discomfort is a part of life and it's OK to be uncomfortable. When I recognize danger in my life, I take the appropriate steps to eliminate it. I stop using food as a "quick fix" for uncomfortable situations and feelings

5) I seek true reassurance for my fears.

I acknowledge my fears and I give myself the reassurance I need for them. I reassure myself with words, actions, and support from others. I am finished using food as a means to hide my fears or as a substitute for comfort, care, and love. Food is only for nourishment, fuel, and to keep my body healthy.

6) Fat is necessary for the health of my body, but too little or too much is unhealthy.

Although I need some fat for my body to function correctly, too much or too little fat is dangerous to my physical health. When the amount of fat on my body interferes with my health, I acknowledge it as a danger signal and take the steps necessary to change my eating patterns into healthier ones. Eating patterns that result in unhealthy amounts of fat for my body may be an indication of an addictive process. I can use the resources available to end addictive cycles, including medical intervention, addiction counseling, or participation in an ongoing support group.

7) I distinguish between food restrictions for physical health and physical image.

My goal is a healthy *body* rather than a two-dimensional body *image*. I stay focused on the reality of what my body tells me rather than the fantasy of ads, media, and societal messages. I respect my body's messages by eliminating foods and eating patterns that hurt me. I gain control of my eating by giving up trying to control the uncontrollable.

8) I trust myself.

As I continue to pay more attention to my body's messages, my focus becomes more personal. I listen to and respect the messages my body sends me. I accept that my body's needs may be totally different from another's. I welcome the eating patterns and program that are healthiest for me.

9) I take care of myself.

I take the time needed to keep an accepting personal environment around me. I treat myself with patience and kindness. I am gentle with myself. I affirm myself with encouraging messages on a daily basis. I deserve only the best. I enjoy taking care of my body in every way possible.

10) I can cope.

I am able to face any challenge that comes along by feeling my own power and knowing I will make a decision that is the right one for me. I don't have to hide behind food anymore because I know now that by using food inappropriately, I cover up my true power. I feel my own strength and will cope as best as I am able with no unrealistic judgments on myself as a person. I look for and learn appropriate ways to cope, and I ask for help when I need it.

11) I stay connected.

I continually check in with myself on whether I am becoming isolated or not. Time by and for myself is important, but when I distance myself personally and spiritually from who and what is helpful, I set myself up for returning to old, unhealthy patterns. Those times that feel the most difficult for me are the times I most need to reconnect.

12) I am OK.

I know that whatever happens, I have people in my life who care about me, and who accept me as the human being I am. I will do no less for myself. I am not "bad" if I make a mistake, nor "good" if I do something well. I acknowledge all the parts of my humanness, including emotions, needs, strengths and weaknesses, and I rejoice in my individuality. Knowing I am OK brings me a peace of mind that enables me to enjoy myself and my life.

13) I renew my commitment on a daily basis.

Today, my commitment is to myself and what is healthiest for me. I acknowledge and accept the eating patterns and foods that are dangerous for me, and remain committed to their elimination. I will do whatever it takes to continue in this commitment. My health and well-being are of primary importance because I want to do more than survive -- I want to live my life with an attitude of gratefulness, optimism, and hope.

These personally affirming messages are suggestions for filling up the hole left behind after eliminating the old messages that have kept you from listening to and respecting your own body about food and eating. Some of the concepts (such as the differences between discomfort and danger, and giving yourself reassurance for your fears), may be unfamiliar right now, but they will be explained more fully in the next chapter.

Rebellion: Healthy or Unhealthy?

Rebellion is one response to those old messages many people experience. It is a way for people to shrug off the rules and restrictions that have been forced onto them by others. Rebellion can take two forms: healthy rebellion and unhealthy rebellion. The type you choose makes the difference between becoming true to your body's messages or remaining connected to the messages others have placed on you.

The authority represented by those old food and eating messages may have felt comfortable in some ways. It has told you what to do, when and how to do it, and when to stop. This is similar to the adult authority you experienced as a child at home, in school, in your religious upbringing, during camp, etc. This type of authority may have been important when you *were* a child in order to teach you guidelines for living, but it only keeps you feeling *like* a child now that you are an adult.

Rebellion is an attempt to assert one's own power and individuality, acknowledging that it may be different from that of the authority. Rebelling in order to get in touch with what is best for you and with your body's messages is healthy. It is important to reclaim your individual power, and healthy rebellion is the means to doing so.

However, when you rebel just to do the opposite of what you're told, the rebellion becomes unhealthy. When you rebel in order to "show" someone you don't have to do what they say, you usually end up hurting yourself. When you rebel because you are rejecting what someone stands for or believes in, you continue to remain focused on that person and their beliefs instead of your own body and what is best for it.

Unhealthy rebellion is the behavior of a child rather than that of an adult. In the areas of food and eating, for example, you may decide to rebel against your parents' messages to "Eat!" by starving or purging; or you may rebel against the image diet's messages to "Don't eat!" by overeating or eating unhealthy foods. You might rebel against your partner because of expectations in the relationship. You might rebel against societal messages because you don't believe you can ever attain such impossible standards. In essence, you don't care what your behavior does to you as long as it is the opposite of what is expected by others.

Healthy rebellion means acting in your own best interest, even though others may have told you differently. You aren't rebelling *because* of what someone else says or believes in, you are rebelling *in order to* discover what's healthiest for you.

Eliminating the messages that have prevented you from being true to yourself is a form of healthy rebellion. You are questioning what those messages have meant for you and making a personal decision about which ones are best for you. This type of rebellion is a sign of self-care. It signals a shift from being overly concerned about what others want for you to being focused on what's actually best for you. It indicates a transition into a new area of personal growth and exploration. This is a very important step in the process of reclaiming your individual power as an adult.

Rebellion is an important part of growth in our lives. During the time known as the "terrible two's," the child is in a state of rebellion. Children rebel against the old messages of babyhood because they are ready to be mobile, communicating kids. Now that the two-year-old can walk and talk, they go exploring in order to find out more about the world around, what the new rules and consequences are, and how they fit in that world.

Another time of rebellion is adolescence. This is a time of leaving childhood behind and preparing for a place in the adult world. Adolescents push on the old messages, eliminate the ones that don't work for them, and attempt to find their places as newly emerging adults with adult responsibilities and consequences.

Healthy rebellion is, in essence, a time of transition. During this time you are attempting to find your place in the new life you are moving toward. Unhealthy rebellion, however, prevents you from making the choices you truly want. It's like spinning your wheels in the mud. Although you want to go forward, the more you try to move ahead, the more you stay where you are, and the deeper you get stuck.

While it may be important to rebel, it is also important to acknowledge that some of the messages you've received *have* been helpful -- the ones that told you about nutrition and health. When you rebel in a healthy manner, you replace only the unhealthy messages with those that are true *to* you and *for* you. You keep the messages about food and eating that promote your health and well-being.

The messages listed here can be used to that extent, or you can create your own. Either way, what's important is that you begin to incorporate these new messages into your life on a daily basis. By reading them to yourself daily, you will continue to promote self-acceptance while keeping the door open to listen to and respect personal messages from your body.

If you have been eating or refusing to eat as an act of unhealthy rebellion, do some exploring in order to determine who or what you have been rebelling against. If you need to rebel, pick and choose ways that won't hurt you. Once you do, you can follow your own rules and establish your own control according to your body's needs.

Obsession, Compulsion, and Addiction

The concepts of obsession, compulsion, and addiction can be extremely confusing for people, and it's important to understand not only their differences, but how they interact with each other. After all, it's the interaction of these three that can cause you to eat when you swore up and down you weren't going to.

Obsession is the thought process that invades and pervades your mind about food and eating. A food and eating obsession has you *thinking* about food most of the time: what you're going to have for your next meal, what you're going to serve your friends or family when they come over, making sure you will have more than enough food when you go camping, wondering if there will be enough food or the kinds of food you like served at the party you're planning to attend, etc. The thought of food and eating is a constant companion. You wonder and worry about whether you will or won't eat at any given time.

Obsession is something that is difficult to overcome, but not impossible. One way to take control of obsessive thinking is to allot one-half hour per day to think about food and eating. Make your plans, worry, wonder -- but do so during a scheduled half hour each day. You may want to select a time in the evening in order to think about what will happen the following day, or in the morning when you take the dog for a walk. Whatever time is best for you is what counts, as long as you remember to only think or worry about food and eating during that specific time. The rest of your day is to think about how you're going to enjoy the rest of the day.

Compulsion is the behavior process that finds you *doing* just the opposite of what you wanted to do <u>without thinking</u> about it. When you feel compelled to do something, you acknowledge a craving or an urge that seems to have no logic or sense about it. It feels overwhelming and you believe you have to give in to it. You believe you have no choice. A compulsion seems to strip you of your sense of power and control.

One reason you give in to a compulsion is because you've taken the focus off yourself. When you lose sight of what your body is saying, you give up your sense of power and control. On the other hand, when you are able to remember how you will feel later, after indulging your compulsion now, you often find the strength to resist.

When you make a commitment to do whatever it takes *not* to eat in ways that are unhealthy for you or that go against your body's messages, you take back your power of choice. When you are committed to utilizing other options such as talking to someone, writing about your feelings, or getting out of the situation that has set up the compulsion, you stay focused on your objective of doing what's healthiest for you. This is one way to resist compulsions and retain control of your eating.

Addiction contains both obsessive and compulsive components. Although some experts say that you can only be addicted to chemical substances that cause changes in your brain, others maintain that anything you do over and over, even though it's continually self-destructive and personally damaging, has an addictive dynamic to its pattern.

Addictions are often characterized by thinking or saying to yourself "I don't ever want to do *that* again," and soon finding yourself doing exactly the same thing. You know what you are doing is not good for you because your body tells you it feels terrible, yet it's not too long before you are making excuses for or justifying the same behavior, hoping somehow the results will be different this time.

Addictions defy logic, knowledge, control, or willpower. They have nothing to do with intelligence or strength. In fact, the more you try to control an addiction, the more you will find yourself defeated. It's only by acknowledging this is something that cannot be controlled do you have a chance of putting an addiction into remission. This is the essence of the statement in the list of personal messages that says: "The only way to control the uncontrollable is to give up trying to control it." The assignment at the end of this chapter will help you to recognize and identify any possible out-of-control food and eating areas that you may have.

Binge Eating and Stockpiling

Binge eating is often done out of a sense of feeling deprived. It is usually connected with the idea of dieting or "should/shouldn't" eating. Usually the idea of dieting includes looking ahead to a period of time in which you are not allowed to eat your favorite foods (before going on a diet) or looking back on a period of time in which you were denied your favorite foods (after just finishing a diet). "Should/shouldn't" eating includes the belief about what is or isn't allowed for you to eat at any given time.

Binge eating is a way to make up for the feeling of being deprived of the foods you really want. You binge on foods in order to make up for what you have been or will be missing, and you give yourself permission to do so because you believe it is the way to feel satisfied.

Many people binge right after they've finished a diet. You've attained your goal, the diet is over, and now is the time to reward yourself for passing up all those hot fudge sundaes or banana cream pies, or for feeling half-starved for the past six months. Feeling deprived from giving up what you want and believe you deserve sets you up for a binge.

Feeling powerless to resist what's in the refrigerator or freezer either at home or at the store, yet knowing you should resist/shouldn't eat all that fattening stuff, and being terrified of getting fat yourself, may set you up for a binge/purge dynamic. In all these instances, feelings of shame, self-hate, and self-anger as well as physical discomfort often accompany the binge. You wish you hadn't done it, and you often find it more difficult to return to healthy, self-focused eating.

Changing your focus and perception of foods from feeling deprived (because you can't have what you want) to wanting what is healthiest for your body, usually helps to eliminate the craving for a binge. Psychotherapy may be necessary, especially to help break a binge/purge cycle and to shatter the overwhelming fear of getting fat. Replacing your "want" list of foods from what your mouth wants to what your body wants often eliminates the feeling of deprivation. It is possible to make binge eating a thing of the past.

A personal example of deprivation eating happened to me over one holiday season. I had never been much of a chocolate eater, but I suddenly felt that I had been deprived of the pleasures of chocolate I'd heard so much about from others. To set this straight (I thought) I bought myself a box of assorted goodies and set about eating as much as I could get my hands on.

I noticed in the back of my mind that none of these candies really tasted as good as I kept expecting them to taste, and that they were upsetting my stomach -- but I didn't let those awarenesses stop me from stuffing my face! I believed that eventually I'd get that chocolate "high" I'd heard about, so I ignored what my body was telling me and kept eating.

I woke up on New Year's Day suddenly realizing that I didn't want chocolate in my life anymore. I felt like I finally allowed myself to be in reality. I accepted that not only didn't chocolate candies taste the way I wanted them to taste, but they weren't doing me any good physically, either. I felt sad. I could admit I had felt deprived of the candy because of the whole aura around chocolate. So many other people thought chocolate was the greatest thing on earth, so I believed I should, too. *Their* messages were interfering with *my* reality!

I don't feel deprived of chocolate anymore because I allowed myself to have it when I thought I wanted it, but I do feel that it is a past part of my life and I can live more enjoyably without it. Even now, when that old tug comes along telling me that I "should" want a heart-shaped box of chocolates, I am able to remember my personal reality and I keep on walking. And that feels good.

Stockpiling is eating in anticipation of food deprivation. Many people stockpile the day before they start a diet. Sundays or New Year's Eve's see a lot of this type of behavior. When you are looking forward to a grim prospect of endless days without your favorite goodies, it makes it hard to resist one last eating orgy. You tell yourself that this will get you through all those barren days of salads and low-fat foods.

An example of stockpiling came from a friend of mine who went through a weight-loss program that required a weekly weigh-in. For most of the week she quite carefully adhered to the diet plan. Immediately after the weigh-in she headed for her favorite ice cream stand for a jumbo hot fudge sundae.

When I asked her about it, she told me that all week she thought about having that hot fudge sundae because it wasn't allowed any more. She knew she'd have to weigh herself in another week, so she had the sundae in order to gear herself up for another week of dieting. Unfortunately, after she reached her goal weight, she began having hot fudge sundaes more often. She told me she was making up for lost time and that she deserved them because she had done so well on her diet program. She regained all the weight she had lost, and then some, within the year.

When you feel deprived of your favorite foods from past diets, and believe you will be deprived again as another diet looms in the near future, the feeling of deprivation sets you up to eat in a non-natural way. Your awareness of your body's messages becomes nonexistent because you are focused on your feeling of deprivation. You eat without thinking what it means to not only your body, but your own sense of well-being because a non-natural belief system has been created. This belief system causes an artificial impression of a dynamic known as supply and demand.

Artificial Supply and Demand

True self-caring is being true to yourself about your hunger, about whether and what kind of food is available, and about allowing yourself to eat what your body needs. When you care for yourself, you do what is best for you now, not to make up for past denial or guard against future unavailability.

The goal of this program is to cultivate and keep a natural belief system around you in order to promote natural eating. A non-natural belief system either works from the past or tries to control the future. Either way, it doesn't look at the "now" of your personal reality. Instead, it helps to set up a situation of artificial supply and demand concerning food and eating.

When you are on a numbers-based diet, your food supply is arti-

HOW TO MAKE PEACE WITH FOOD

ficially restricted. What I mean by artificially is that in reality, if you look at the supply of food available to you, there is little or no limit. There is still plenty of chocolate cake on the grocer's shelves, lots of pizza deliveries available. You only need to hand over the payment.

However, because of the dictates of your diet, you believe there are restraints in effect, and you don't believe you have access to as much cake or pizza as you may be hungry for. This sets up an **artificially** restricted supply, produced from a non-natural belief system. And along with this artificial restriction comes fear.

This fear manifests itself in non-natural behaviors. In the 1970's, there was a threatened gasoline shortage, and everyone was afraid they wouldn't be able to get enough gas. People waited in lines that were hours long because their tanks were only 3/4 full. They did things they didn't normally do for fear of not having all the gas they wanted.

A similar phenomenon happened in the 80's with a certain brand name doll. Just as with gas rationing, when the supply is short, the demand increases. Because there was a restricted supply of dolls, and so many people wanted them, the demand for them was amazingly high. What resulted were stampedes on stores that advertised getting in a new shipment, and people went to great lengths—including stealing from children—in order to have one of those dolls.

The point here is that what you want and aren't allowed to have sets up a high demand type of belief system. Now, because you can't have it, you want it even more; you may even go to great lengths to take more than you really need just to have it, for fear that you might not be able to get it again if you want it later. This is how an artificial supply sets up an artificial demand.

The same phenomenon can happen with food. When the supply of what you want is cut off in an artificial manner, such as through numbers-based diets, your demand for it goes up in an artificial way. Suddenly, it's all you want, and you do things that feel out of control, like stockpiling and binge eating. This is how you eat from fear rather than from hunger.

This environment of artificial supply and demand has set you up to be out of control with your hunger. You've eaten from fear of deprivation in the future because of experiencing deprivation in the past, rather than actual hunger in the present. And because you didn't know that you have the power to eat whatever you want when you are hungry for it, you did what you were set up to do: you ate non-naturally.

Since everyone's body experience is different, it only follows that everyone's eating patterns are, too. Each person will be hungry at different times, for different foods, and for different amounts of those foods. One person may eat at 9:00 a.m. and not be hungry again for 3 or 4 more hours, while another person may eat at 9:00 a.m. and be hungry again at 10:00 a.m. Some people eat small amounts of food several times throughout the day, while others are more comfortable eating only 2 or 3 times each day. Eating patterns are as individual as the person.

Stress Relief – Distracting Yourself with Food

You may have already learned through therapy, weight-loss programs, or even magazine articles, that you often eat because you are lonely, anxious, angry, etc., rather than hungry. Because certain emotions or situations make you uncomfortable, you have learned to relieve the stress of that discomfort with food. However, even though in the past you may have used food to make yourself feel better, you are also realizing that it's not making you feel better anymore.

Eating for relief or escape is a difficult cycle to break. Food doesn't change the situation you are in nor does it make your emotions go away, but you don't know what else to do. This can make for a lot of confusion and a lot of negative thinking. There's nothing wrong with you; your belief system has been programmed to keep false hopes and unrealistic expectations alive. Part of getting out of such a cycle is changing that belief system to reflect the reality of yourself and your life.

Tackling those beliefs takes time, determination, and energy. Unlike quick-fix methods, the goal here is to do what is best for *you* in your life. Learning what needs to be done gives you the opportunity to continue traveling in the direction of healthy behaviors and beliefs. As you start making the decisions that are healthiest for yourself, you will find you get filled up from within. You will begin to feed yourself what it is you are really hungry for.

At this point in your life, however, you may be regularly feeding yourself food to ease stress rather than hunger. You do this because it is what you know how to do. You have learned to eat in order to make your life more comfortable for yourself. Your stress reliever for life's slings and arrows are in your kitchen or at a fast-food drive-thru. Food is what you count on to get you through the uncomfortable times of your life.

It's important to put food in its proper perspective. Food, itself, is like electricity. Electricity can kill you or it can enhance your life; it all depends on how it's used. Just because it can kill you doesn't mean you must stop using it altogether. It's the same with food. Chocolate cake isn't good or bad--it would be pretty difficult to live on cake alone, but then it would be pretty difficult to live for long on lettuce alone, as well. Food is simply food.

Along with body messages about what *kinds* of food are needed, your body also tells you how much of each kind it wants. Your body will tell you what you need to know if you just listen to it. Because listening to your body's messages may be a new concept for you, you may feel a bit of anxiety or fear. If you haven't been used to listening to your body and its messages, you may even feel skeptical that it will communicate with you at all. It takes time and practice to know your body won't let you down.

This practice is no different than the practice it takes to play a Mozart concerto on the piano. When you first sit down before the keys, you may be anxious, thinking you'll never be able to do this. Looking at the keys and the music may feel overwhelming. You don't know how to place your fingers, you don't know how to read notes, you may have performance anxiety and you're sure that everything will turn out rotten. But through lessons, and practice, you gradually see results. It takes a willingness to learn something new and a determination to keep at it until you get it.

And just like faltering at the piano while first learning the piece, you will also falter in your new ways of eating. You won't be perfect at this, but you will continue to get to a place where this new way is more and more comfortable to you, where you rely on food less for stress and comfort and more for fuel.

As this happens, your focus will be less on weight-- and the less it is on weight, the more your focus will be on your body and what it is saying to you. You will find your weight will take care of itself and won't be a major concern of yours. When this begins to happen, you will be living a happier, more peaceful life where food is concerned. One more battle will be whittled away.

When you eat just what you want and the amount of food that fits in your stomach at that time, you will know that it agrees with you and your body. If you have ever experienced this type of eating, you know that it happens when you eat just what you are hungry for, you enjoy eating it, and you stop at just the right time, before you are stuffed to distraction. You think to yourself "Wow, that really hit the spot!"

That's what you're aiming for here--to consistently eat in this manner. The food will have tasted good right down to the last bite, and then it will be enough. And that's one way to tell if the food is right for you--it will taste good. When it doesn't taste good anymore, it's either not what you really want, or it's more than you really want. It's just another message from your body to be listened to.

Our Image of Fat

It's amazing how much negative press there has been about fat, yet we need fat for our bodies to run efficiently. Nutritionists will tell you that fat soluble vitamins aren't available to be used by our bodies without fat. Women's bodies especially need a certain percentage of fat or they stop menstruating. A compulsive runner friend of mine was on special medication to bring her period back. It stopped because of the lack of body fat she had.

This is not "normal" in a very physical sense for our bodies. There are many reports of athletic women being anorexic or bulimic because the emphasis is on weight, or more precisely, on carrying less weight than their body would normally hold. In a non-natural situation, you will eat non-naturally. With a non-natural emphasis, you will eat non-naturally. When your focus is in a more natural place, you will eat more naturally.

Weekly Assignment

This leads us to your assignment for this chapter. The first part of it I already mentioned--make a list of your new personal messages and put them somewhere so that you will be able to see and read them every day. It may be on your refrigerator, on your desk at the office, on the visor of your car, or on the mirror in your bedroom.

The second part of your assignment is to keep a chart of your eating for a week. Before you moan and groan about keeping a food chart, this one is different. This chart is for trouble-shooting. As you keep track of what you're eating and why, you will begin to become aware of problem areas of control that you might not have noticed in the past.

Turn to the Appendix, Page (viii), the chart labeled *Trouble-shooting*. To fill out the chart, begin in the first column, marked "Food," and write down the kind of food you are eating. In the second column, marked "Reason for Eating," write down why you are eating that particular food. Some reasons may be for hunger, because you're nervous, because you're bored, because it's a habit while watching TV, or whatever your particular reason is.

The third column, marked "Did/Didn't Stop," is the one that will give you information about whether or not you are in control. This column is designed to allow you to get into reality about stopping when you know it's best to stop, or continuing on in spite of what you know is best. You are not expected to change anything right now, just to become aware of where you may be out of control.

The fourth column, marked "Meaning for Food," invites you to look for the *underlying* meaning for your eating, or for the particular food you picked. Different from the reason that you're eating, this column is looking for what your food and eating represents for you at this particular time. For example, if your reason for eating is hunger, and you eat food that is nourishing, the meaning for the food would be fuel. If the reason for your eating is boredom, the meaning for eating might be "something to do." However, you picked a certain type of food to eat, and that particular kind of food might represent something special. If you're eating because you're anxious, the food might represent something your mom gave you to calm you or comfort you.

The more information you put into these columns, the more information you will have to work with when you get into the next chapter about comforting yourself with food. This chart will give you a lot of knowledge that will be useful for you in understanding why you eat what you eat when you eat it.

To Remember

- Old messages have power over you when you don't believe you have adult choices about food and eating
- Rebellion is a time of transition, moving from what you accepted without question to a place of new rules, experiences, and consequences
- Healthy rebellion encourages questioning what went on before and making choices that enhance your life no
- Obsession is the constant thinking about something; compulsion is doing something without thought of the consequences; addiction contains components of both these dynamics
- Binge eating and stockpiling are forms of eating for feelings of deprivation in the past and anticipation of deprivation for the future
- The type of commitment you make influences the decisions you make regarding your food and eating choices. The type of commitment you make reflects how much you are emotionally ready and able to risk
- Each person moves at their own rate of readiness

CHAPTER IV

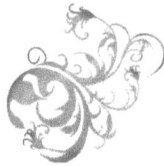

COMFORTING OURSELVES

Assignment Review

Assignment 1

The first assignment was to read the list of positive personal messages on a daily basis. These new messages are a way to fill the void left after eliminating the old, unhealthy messages that were part of the work accomplished in Chapter III. Any void demands to be filled. You have the choice of refilling this void with new, healthy messages for yourself, or letting the void be, in which case, it will refill itself. The problem with letting it be is that it can only refill itself with the kinds of messages you have been familiar with in the past. Without conscious effort, the negative will creep back in, and you'll find yourself back in that vicious lose/gain cycle once more.

Most of those old messages served to keep you farther and farther out of touch with your body and its messages to you, while the new, healthier messages allow room for communication with your body and encourage you to listen to and respect what it's telling you. This is how you re-establish a sense of self-acceptance and self-trust. It will take time; you have had many years of practice ignoring and denying your body and what it says to you. As you continue to practice, your body's messages will become clearer, you will hear them more easily, and eventually you will make healthier, more natural choices in the foods you eat and in how you eat them.

Assignment 2

The second assignment from Chapter III included keeping a week-long chart of foods and eating patterns in order to become more aware of where your own particular trouble areas are. Trouble areas are the times in which or the foods with which you don't stop eating, even though you know you're hurting yourself or you're not being true to your body's messages. These are the areas where you're out of control, the areas that have caused you pain, frustration, anger, despair, and even self-loathing. These are the areas during which you find excuses to hurt yourself with food, the times you use food for something other than fuel.

Think about feeling out of control, what it means to be out of control. It means that no amount of trying, willpower, determination, intelligence, or strength will stop it from happening again. You have been attempting to control the uncontrollable. Trying to control the uncontrollable is the basis for an addiction dynamic.

The Addiction Connection

Whether your out-of-control areas have been a type of food (such as chocolate, bread, sweets, ice cream, chips, fast food, etc.), certain times for eating (when you're alone, at night, after work, on breaks, feeling stressed, etc.), or during certain situations (at parties, in a restaurant, on vacation, during a holiday, etc.), these are the times during which you have given yourself permission to hurt yourself with food. This permission constitutes the essence of an addictive component.

The charting exercise can help you become aware of the foods and situations with which you hurt yourself through eating, and can offer you an indication of the possibility of an addictive process at work. It is not my job, nor within my power to say if you actually are addicted to food. You are the only one who can make that call. However, the idea of hurting yourself over and over with food, either by eating too much or too little of it, and not stopping such behavior even when you know it's hurting you, is strongly indicative of an addictive process.

An addiction, by its very nature, denotes uncontrollable behaviors, distorted thinking, and attempts at control. For many of us, the idea of being out of control with something is unacceptable. We have learned that it's important to be in control at all times. These, then, become the un-successful attempts at controlling our eating patterns and behaviors, which invariably lead us to feeling frustrated, weak, angry at ourselves, stupid, and failures.

Control issues are some of the most difficult to face. We've been taught to not only keep ourselves under control, but our situations and the lives of those around us as well. In truth, the only thing in our lives over which we have control is ourselves: our way of looking at the world, our attitudes, how we react to our emotions, how we deal with situations, how we relate to others, and how we accomplish being the person we want to be.

The rest is out of our control. We can't control how another person feels, what lies around the corner, what people think of us, or how life will treat us. The only thing in your life you can control is yourself.

An example of this comes from personal experience. During the course of a program I was teaching, I planned to postpone one group meeting because I would be out of town. Since we had been meeting on a weekly basis for six weeks by this time, the group had become part of the members' routine. When I told the participants we wouldn't be having a group the following week, most of them expressed feelings of dismay, because this part of their routine had become enjoyable to them. One group member, however, expressed a completely different feeling. She was glad we wouldn't be meeting the following week because, she, too, would be out of town, and had been afraid she was going to have to miss that group.

This experience showed me the truth of the idea that we can't control other people's feelings. Even though I had spoken the same words, and my action would affect everyone the same way, people had different feelings about it because of their own perspectives of the situation. Your feelings come from your perspective, and you can't ever really know the exact perspective of another person. In the end, you are the only one who knows how you feel about something and the extent and depth of that feeling, and you are the only one who can change your perspective in order to change your feelings.

Your perspective on being out of control regarding food and eating will make it harder or easier for you to do what is necessary to change. For example, because the diabetic's body doesn't assimilate sugar the way other bodies do, it's how the diabetic deals with the situation that will make their life either healthier and more enjoyable, or the opposite. Depending on the perspective a diabetic has for this situation, they can choose to accept such a condition and work within it, or continually fight against it, trying to control what is uncontrollable.

Similarly, how you choose to look at the fact of being out of control with aspects of food choices and eating behaviors, you will either continue a self-destructive battle, or acknowledge and admit there is a problem out of your control. To accept this is the first step in leaving the battle behind and winning the war.

To stop trying to control the uncontrollable is what opens the door to doing what is truly appropriate for your situation. For the diabetic, accepting that sugar is off limits because it is dangerous allows the diabetic to do what they need to do to get on with having a happier, healthier life. In the case of your own food choices and eating behaviors, the same concept works.

Once again I will suggest the idea of attending an Overeaters' Anonymous group, (designed to address any types of unhealthy eating patterns, including starving, binging, and purging) where the first step of that program is admitting you are powerless over food, and that your life has become unmanageable. If you have been battling and losing in your war to control your eating habits, you know what unmanageable feels like.

Letting Go of "Trying"

It was Yoda who said "Do. Or do not. There is no try." Another phrase says "Trying is lying." The idea of trying to do something is, in actuality, a failed attempt. The way to stop this failing is to stop trying. This is where elimination can provide relief. In essence, the only way to take control of the uncontrollable is to give up trying to control it. It's by eliminating the hurtful and unhealthy behaviors and food you have tried to control without success that you also eliminate the frustration and failure that accompanies the "trying."

The diabetic who decides to alter their diet by eliminating sugar chooses to accept the reality of their body and stops trying to control the way it responds to sugar. The same thing happens when someone who experiences the dynamic of an addictive process chooses to eliminate their out-of-control foods and behaviors. When these are eliminated due to the acceptance of the fact that to continue them will only persist in hurting you, you are making a conscious decision to eliminate something harmful from your life through personal choice rather than from a sense of "I have to", "I can't", or "I should/shouldn't."

The importance of choice cannot be overemphasized. Choice is personal, conscious, and powerful. Choice is a decision made through your own sense of what's best for you. You are the only one responsible for your choices, and you are the only one who truly realizes the consequences, both positive and negative. It's changing through choice that alters your perspective and gives you a newfound sense of strength to maintain both the choice and the change.

I've often challenged clients to "try" to untie a shoelace. Of course, each one accomplished the untying. At that point I remarked that I had told them only to "try" to untie the shoelace. After a few seconds of puzzled looks, everyone then understood that you either do it or you don't. "Trying" doesn't make it happen.

Similarly, you either do it or you don't when it comes to an addictive or self-destructive behavior. The alcoholic doesn't give up drinking, per se, only stops drinking alcoholic beverages. The gambling addict doesn't stop using money, only stops betting with it. The workaholic doesn't have to stop working, just needs to eliminate working past healthy boundaries.

So, too, for a person who has a problem with food choices and eating behaviors. You don't have to give up eating food, you only need to eliminate the eating patterns and food choices that hurt you. For example, if you found you overeat when you go to a fast-food place, you eliminate going to those places. If you discovered you overeat when it comes to salty, crunchy foods such as chips, you eliminate buying/eating those particular foods. If you now know that you can't eat just one chocolate, you refuse the first one, just like an alcoholic refuses the first drink. It's by eliminating that first "grab" that prevents the second one from happening.

If you are an emotional overeater, support from groups, talking to helpful friends, learning more about how to deal directly with emotionally-charged situations, or changing your perspective, perhaps with professional help, in order to change your emotions, can help eliminate the underlying urge to eat in an unhealthy manner. It's totally personal, totally individual, and totally self-focused. If what you've been doing up till now has been working for you, by all means keep doing it. If it hasn't, however, maybe it's time to look at what hasn't been working, accept that "trying" to control what you've been doing hasn't made it happen, and decide it's time to do something different. The choice is up to you.

Beginning the Transition

Identification and acceptance of personal out-of-control areas can be a difficult task. However, they are crucial to making the transition in your food and eating patterns, from unhealthy, non-natural patterns to healthier, more personally-focused choices. This transition includes questioning your old beliefs and perceptions about food and eating, and the part your own attitude plays in all this.

Confusion and frustration are also components of transition. They are signs you are moving and growing. It's important to realize that your old messages, habits, patterns and perceptions have been with you for a long time – and it will take a period of confusion and frustration to sort through them in order to decide what is best for you and what it is you want to change.

Something else to remember is to keep a positive atmosphere around yourself. We grow and learn best in an atmosphere of encouragement, patience, and caring. This is where your positive personal messages can be a tremendous help. While you may have missed out on these kinds of messages in your past, you now have the ability to give them to yourself. You've earned it.

At this point in the program, you may have already started noticing some changes you are making in your food and eating choices. You may also be more aware of the messages your body is giving you, your hunger and full signals, or the messages about which foods agree and disagree with you. You may be more aware of what you're putting in your mouth and why, and when you are using food as something other than fuel. Now is the time to begin exploring how you have used food to nurture yourself emotionally.

A "Scraped Knee"

Understanding why you attempt to nurture yourself with food begins with learning what emotional nurturance actually means. According to the dictionary, nurturance comes from the Latin meaning to nurse. Synonyms include: to nourish, to care for, and to parent. While it's true that you can nourish and care for your body physically with food, too often you also attempt to nourish and care for your emotions, feelings, and spirit (all those intangibles), with food. Attempting to care for and nourish your being with food and eating just doesn't work. It takes more than food to meet the emotional needs of a child, yet many parents or other care-givers haven't known that.

Being a nurturing parent takes time, energy, and understanding. It involves showing care, affection, reassurance, and comfort. It means being there for support and encouragement, affirming the whole person that makes up a child: mentally and emotionally. It means anticipating a problem, going to the heart of it, and giving the child something real and reliable to depend on in times of trouble. Rarely have parents been able to accomplish all this due to work schedules, family duties, lack of knowledge, or just plain exhaustion from dealing with children and other factors of day-to-day living. Besides, no parent is perfect.

Think back to being a child who, for example, has fallen off a bike and scraped a knee. After an injury, children see the blood and feel the pain. They don't have the comprehension, experience, or logic to assess the reality of the situation. All they know is that they hurt, and they're afraid of what that pain means. They've seen others in pain, bleeding, either in real life, on TV, or at the movies, and sometimes it goes very bad for them. When a child is injured, they draw on very limited experience; when a child feels pain, they are afraid of what it might mean for them.

Usually the first thing a child does when experiencing pain and/or fear is to run to a parent or other adult caregiver. This child needs to know they will be all right, and that the adult will take care of them in this painful and frightening situation. Depending on what kind of care you were given in such circumstances, that's how you've learned to care for yourself when you experience pain and/or fear.

If the adults in your life gave you the kind of nurturance you needed for your pain and fear, several things would have happened. During these groups I ask members to call out what they believed they needed when experiencing pain and fear as a child. The most common ones included three parts:

A). Assessing the situation for its severity. The adult would determine if this was a dangerous situation that needed immediate help, such as a broken leg, or simply a scraped knee, which could be taken care of on the spot. One is a danger situation, the other a discomfort situation.

B). Comforting words of reassurance and validation from the adult.

C). Appropriate actions from the adult.

The assessment process determines if the situation can be dealt with as is, or if help is needed. If your leg was broken, a trip to the hospital would be in order. If it's only a scraped knee, cleaning and caring for the wound could be done then and there. Crying would be allowed, because crying is what we do when we're in pain.

During and after the first aid comes words of reassurance and validation for your feelings. Here is where your fear and pain would be acknowledged as natural parts of a personal injury. The adult would tell you with words such as, "I know it hurts, but eventually the pain will go away so that you will want to play with your friends again," or "Are you scared? I get scared when I'm hurt, but don't worry. I'm here and I'll take care of you," or even soothing sounds.

These kinds of words reassure you that you will survive the experience. They let you know the extent of the damage, that there is more discomfort than danger, and that all your feelings are valid. You are acknowledged and affirmed for your own reality, and you learn not only that it's OK to be afraid, but also that someone is there to take care of you.

Appropriate actions include touch, holding, and physical closeness. They let you know you are safe and not alone. We need healthy touch as a way to flourish and to aid with the healing process. Putting an arm around you, giving you a hug, or holding you for a while are all types of touch that can feel good and relay the messages that you are worth time and attention. You feel safe, cared for, and loved.

Assessment, Reassurance, and Comfort

Assessment, reassurance and comfort are the three necessities for dealing with fear and pain. Assessment provides us with the reality of the situation, reassurance lets us know we will survive, and comfort eases the pain. The quality and quantity of each of these that you received from the adults in your life when you were growing up has been the basis for how you assess your own situation, what kind of reassurance you are able to give yourself, and what kind of comfort you feel from knowing you are worth the time and energy needed to make it through whatever situation is at hand, be it physical or emotional.

Assessment, reassurance, and comfort for emotional "bumps and bruises" can be difficult to give yourself. For example, it's easy to see when your knee is scraped. It's easy to recognize you feel physical pain. However, emotional pain may be more difficult to identify. The fear behind the injury may not be as easily recognized, especially if your fears have been ignored, brushed aside, ridiculed, or simply denied.

We all have fears, we all feel pain. It's when our fears and pain haven't been affirmed adequately throughout our lives that we have problems distinguishing, acknowledging, admitting, and accepting them. Without being able to easily recognize your fears and pain, it becomes difficult to make a valid assessment of your situation.

For example, any type of abuse, whether it be physical (being struck in any manner, or even physically threatened), mental (mind games, or anything that makes you doubt yourself, your perceptions, or your feelings), emotional (being made to feel ashamed or afraid of any of your emotions or not being taught how to appropriately express your emotions), sexual (anything inappropriate or unwanted, or witnessing inappropriate behavior) or spiritual abuse (being taught through fear to believe in something, or not being allowed to question belief systems) will automatically make it difficult for you to recognize and acknowledge your pain and fear because you had to submerge them in order to survive the abuse.

Other experiences that can make assessment of a situation difficult include being given too much responsibility at too young an age (the Red Cross won't accept anyone under the age of 11 in their babysitting course), being given inappropriate responsibility (having to assume a parental role to an incapacitated parent), or being forced to be "different" from your peers (due to family, religion, culture, money, or other reasons). Any such situation requires you to deny your emotions and any pain that may accompany them. You are compelled to "put up" with the situation and survive it as best you can without accompanying knowledge or comfort.

The problem becomes one of backlog. As you experienced more and more situations where you had to deny, push down, shove aside, try to ignore, or pretend about yourself and your feelings, especially those of pain and fear, the harder they became to overlook. You began using something to help distract you from those feelings that were crying to get out. Among other things, you began using food and eating as a way to keep from feeling what was really there.

You might have even been introduced to using food and eating by someone who cared about you. "Here, have a cookie, it'll make you feel better." Advertising has gone a long way to foster this belief, and to play on your denial system when it comes to emotions and feelings. Being told there's a "hug in a mug," that "nothin' says lovin' like something from the oven," or that "happiness tastes like . . ." whatever food is being promoted are all marketing ploys that attempt to replace your emotions with food. You've been inundated with information from many sources about how your feelings should and can be changed, and food has been one way to do it.

As you continued to deny your fears and pain, they continued to pile up. As you felt their pressure, you turned more and more to unhealthy food and non-natural eating patterns to ease that pressure and to make the feelings go away. But they didn't leave, and you became more uncomfortable regarding situations that included the feelings of fear and pain.

Eventually, even the thought of these types of situations scared you, and you felt threatened. You became so uncomfortable, you reacted to them as if they were dangerous, and did even more of what you had learned to do to keep those feelings away. You ate, you starved, you binged, you purged, you exercised, you dieted; in essence, you attempted to comfort and reassure yourself you would be safe against the now-perceived danger of your feelings of fear and pain. You were doing what you knew how to do in order to survive.

Discomfort vs. Danger – The Lion's Roar

Assessing a situation means determining if it is merely something uncomfortable, or if there is truly a danger present. By danger, I mean something that threatens your life, be it emotionally, mentally, spiritually, or physically. We will always survive discomfort; it is danger that we must take steps to protect ourselves against. Determining the difference is our real challenge. We have grown up surrounded by so many dangerous

---

situations that it can be difficult to know what is truly dangerous for us, and what is merely uncomfortable.

Anything that threatens our sensation of well-being, our wholeness as a person, our ability to relate to ourselves and others honestly, our sense of values and morals, or our capacity for feeling and appropriately expressing our emotions is dangerous to us. Our feelings themselves are not dangerous because they are a part of us, but they can feel dangerous because of our experiences when we've tried to acknowledge and express them. Feelings are uncomfortable because we haven't had much practice in allowing them without judgment or punishment.

Being who you are is not dangerous to you, although it, too, may feel so. Again, you probably haven't had very much practice in being the real you, and you may even wonder who you really are. The discomfort in being you feels dangerous, however, because of the consequences you experienced when you attempted to be just that in the past. You often weren't taught how to be the best you there is.

It's the things, situations, and people who try to prevent you from feeling your feelings, or being who you truly are, that are the real dangers in your life. You've had to learn how to survive in spite of them when you had no choice. As an adult, now, all that's changed, and you are beginning to feel your own adult power as you begin to take your life back.

One story I heard gives an example of the difference between real and perceived danger. Think about lions in the wild. They hunt in packs, with the females being the hunters for the pride. One way they get help in their hunting is by having one of the older males with a fierce, menacing roar, go to the other side of the field where a herd of game will be coming through. As the prey approaches, the lions take up their positions. The male begins roaring, while the females lie in wait on the opposite side. As the herd gets nearer and hears the roar, it perceives danger, and runs away. Of course, it turns right into the path where the females, the true danger, lie in wait.

This story shows the difference between perceived and real danger, and what they mean for us in our lives. The herd hears the roar of the lion, and becomes afraid, knowing that lions mean death. What the herd mentality doesn't understand is that the roar is only air, and can't really hurt them. That old male lion is no hunter, he just sounds scary, but the herd reacts to the sound as if it were dangerous. It makes them uncomfortable and frightened. When they turn away from it, they are turning away from a perception of danger. They turn instead to where the real danger lies, and death is indeed waiting.

Every scary situation has the possibility of a roar or real danger. Even though it is not dangerous, the roar triggers anxiety and fear because of past experiences. These feelings have become so uncomfortable for you that you perceive them to be unsafe, even life-threatening. Like the herd, you often don't realize the difference between what is uncomfortable and what is actually dangerous.

This is where reality assessment is so important. If you respond to every roar that reminds you of a past situation or person that harmed you, that damaged you, that presented a true threat to you being, you will respond as if you were in true danger once again, and go for a "quick fix." In the story of the lion's roar, the "quick fix" for the herd was to run away from the roar, which led them into the path of the waiting huntress, the true danger. They weren't able to assess the reality of their situation, and turned from that which seemed dangerous to that which was truly dangerous.

In times of true danger, it's necessary to fix the situation as quickly as possible. In times of discomfort, however, it's reassurance and comfort that you need, neither of which are "quick fixes" because both take time and energy. You have "quick fixed" your feelings of discomfort to the roars in your life through food choices, overeating, excess exercise, and/or starving and purging.

These types of behaviors have led you into a place of true danger, that of self-abuse. It's through self-abuse that you have been both physically and emotionally hurting yourself. You've reacted to discomfort as if it were danger, and have been damaging your body and mind in the process. What you've needed, but haven't known how to give to yourself, is reassurance for the fear and anxiety, and comfort for the pain.

Reassurance for our Fears, Comfort for our Pain

Reassurance and comfort are integral parts of dealing with fear and pain, yet they are often absent from our lives. Reassurance lets us know we are able to cope with whatever feels threatening to us, allowing us to work through the fear or anxiety in an appropriate manner. Comfort enables us to bear whatever pain we may be feeling by giving us the strength to know the pain won't overwhelm us and that we will make it through.

Reassurance and comfort are often concepts that are unknown to us. They include feelings of affection which let us know we are cared about, and empowerment, which lets us experience a sense of personal courage in the face of adversity. Reassurance and comfort also provide us with the realization that we can ask for help if we aren't able to cope with a situation on our own. They enable us to withstand the discomfort and know we will survive the experience. There is no shame, blame or guilt involved, only acknowledgment of our fears, and the strength to do what is appropriate for the circumstances.

Reassurance and comfort are part of a process freely given that allays our fears and lets us know we are safe. Unfortunately, the reassurance and comfort we have needed throughout our lives has often been absent or confounded by unknowing adults. That which we haven't experienced for ourselves is difficult to give to ourselves.

Our greatest fear is that we will not be able to cope with a situation, and our deepest pain is the shame we feel at failing to cope. Your perceptions of what any person or situation may mean to you is what set you up for your fear and/or anxiety, and your anticipation of the pain that may accompany it. If, as a child, you were forced into a situation that was beyond your ability to cope, yet you were expected to cope with it as an adult would, then any present situation similar to the past can trigger both that fear and pain you originally experienced.

Any situation where you believed you could not or were not allowed to say "no," were forced to do something against your will because you were too afraid not to, or were coerced into doing something that didn't feel good to you can trigger you in the present. Similar situations, people, circumstances, smells, environments, pictures – anything that may remind you of a past hurt – can be a trigger for an automatic "danger" feeling, no matter how truly safe and far away from the original situation you are.

It's your perception of the situation or the person that triggers your fear, not the reality. The reality was in the past, but the fear and pain were so great that they color your present and future. Because you weren't able to keep yourself safe at some time in your past, you believe you won't be able to keep yourself safe now. This can encourage you to use food and eating as an ally to help bury or distract you from the fear and pain, and hopefully to prevent a reoccurrence of that which scared and hurt you.

Using food and eating in this manner is your way to "quick fix" your perception of being in danger. Without confronting this fear and rendering it powerless in your life, you will continue to feel as if you're in danger when you hear a "roar" from the past. When your fear has been confronted and resolved, you might still feel uncomfortable when a "roar" rears its shaggy head, but you'll be aware that you can now assess the situation for its reality, take the steps necessary to comfort yourself in a meaningful manner, and leave food and eating to their rightful places as fuel for your body.

Discomfort vs. Danger

The inability to discern between discomfort and true danger causes you to believe that discomfort is the same as danger. Danger needs to be fixed as soon as possible, while discomfort needs reassurance and comforting until the discomfort passes. This difference is vital to your sense of well-being and confidence.

Rarely have we learned how to assess a situation for the difference between discomfort and danger. In the scraped knee example, your pain told you something was wrong, and that scared you, but you didn't have the knowledge or experience to assess the true extent of what was wrong by yourself. You may have had an idea, but when we're kids, our logic and knowledge are limited. We know what we feel, but we're not sure it's "right." We turned to an adult for the assessment, and believed that adult's messages, even if they differed from our own.

If that adult told you, with or without words, to ignore the pain and/or the fear, or that some type of behavior or substance would help "fix" the situation, you did what you were told. You ate the cookie or ice cream or pizza and became distracted or full, or maybe even overfull, but you discovered that the pain/fear didn't bother you as much. Such behavior, repeatedly used, became habit, and in the process, you learned how to ignore or bury your feelings and body's messages.

In this manner, you began to automatically "fix" every discomfort with an outside substance and/or an inappropriate behavior. You never learned how to assess a situation or feeling for danger, and often stayed in dangerous situations trying to fix them or your feelings about them with food and eating behaviors. You learned to distrust your feelings and your body's messages; in the process, you learned to distrust yourself. You were never taught how to realistically assess a situation for its danger potential and began responding to many of your feelings in the same way.

If you felt afraid, nervous, anxious, you ate. If you felt sad, you ate If you felt angry, you ate. If you felt happy, you ate to celebrate. Your first priority for company coming over was to make sure you had enough food. Your first priority when visiting was wondering if there would be food there.

What you didn't do was identify your feeling, assess the situation for its danger potential, and give yourself the reassurance you needed to make it through an uncomfortable experience. Because of what you weren't taught, you never learned you were capable of coping with a situation in the manner healthiest and most appropriate for you and the circumstances. This left you with a hole where the reassurance belonged, and you only knew to try to fill that hole with food.

You began to routinely cover your discomfort, chase it away, or deny its existence with food and eating behaviors. You detached yourself from the discomfort by focusing on food and/or some type of non-natural eating pattern, or exercise regimen. By focusing on weight and body image issues, you buried and denied your emotions and your discomfort and filled yourself with self-doubt instead.

Eating, not eating, exercise, and purging all became ways to defend yourself against the discomfort of emotions and situations. These defense mechanisms helped you to feel in control of your emotions, your situation, your life, and yourself, even as you were feeling more and more out of control. For a while they may have seemed to work; you were distracted, you were able to ignore, to pretend, to bury, to look the other way, to give yourself a false sense of security and control, or even to laugh things off.

However, you've come to the point in your life where you realize it isn't working anymore. Your fears are still there, bigger than ever. You feel more out of control, like you're spiraling downward. You may even be in physical danger now due to food and eating abuse. Now may be the time to face your fears, learning how to acknowledge and deal with them in a more appropriate manner. To do this, it's important to explore the part fear plays in your sense of being happy.

Fear – The Bottom Line

Remember those word games that asked you to move from one word to a totally different word in a certain number of moves by changing one letter in each succeeding word? This is a sequence I've discovered that works something like that. It moves you, starting at the bottom and moving upward, from the feeling of fear to the feeling of happiness. Each step in this ladder is based on acknowledging and completing the step before:

Happiness
Making Personal Choices
Feeling Empowered/Self-Confident
Having a Positive Sense of Self-Worth
Feeling Safe
Assessment/Reassurance/Comfort
Fear

The bottom line is fear - the fear of getting hurt, the fear of pain, the fear of not being taken care of, the fear of dying. I believe fear is underneath all our non-natural perspectives, attitudes, and responses in any given situation, either real or perceived. When you are able to acknowledge and identify why you are afraid, and get the reassurance needed for the fear, anxiety, worry, or nervousness you face, you will be able to stop using food inappropriately in your life. Here is the sequence in more detail:

Fear

Your fears (or close cousins, anxiety, worry, and nervousness) and the procedures you choose for dealing with them sets the tone for this entire sequence, and determines whether you will, in general, be a happy or unhappy person. When you are able to accept that sometimes you will feel afraid, acknowledge those times you actually are afraid, and identify what you're afraid of, you can begin to seek the reassurance needed to overcome the fear and put it to rest.

Fear is part of life; everyone feels afraid at one time or another. It is a protective emotion to warn us when danger looms. What is most often connected with fear is pain or getting hurt, emotionally, mentally, sexually, physically, or spiritually. Because of your individual experience with any of these areas, your fears will also be individual as will the intensity of your fears. You are the only one who can affirm them, assess them, and face them. This can be done on your own, with support from friends, family, groups, professionals, or a mix of these. No one knows the intensity of each fear you feel, or how best for you to confront it. That's your call. I always suggest to use everything possible until you get a better grasp of exactly what you face.

It isn't until you name your fears that you can begin to assess for the reality of danger or discomfort. If there is indeed a danger present, you know it's time for fast action. However, if it is only a discomfort you feel, you can reassure yourself you have the ability to deal with the situation. Either way, the fear is put in its rightful place, and will cause less and less of a problem in your life.

Assessment/Reassurance/Comfort

Reassurance is the key to coping with fear. Without reassurance, we have difficulty believing that we can cope with our situation or emotions. We get that reassurance when we are able to assess a situation for its true danger potential. Again, if the situation is truly dangerous, it's imperative that we take quick action to keep ourselves safe. If, however, the situation is only uncomfortable, we know it will soon pass, and we can reassure ourselves it will not harm us. It's up to you to decide if you're dealing with the "lion" or the "roar," and act accordingly.

If you are uncomfortable with your emotions, it may help to write them down or talk to someone about them. Emotions will never harm you because they are a part of you. They may be uncomfortable if you haven't had a lot of practice feeling, acknowledging, or expressing them appropriately. It's in knowing you are able to cope that comforts you and allows you to feel safe.

Feeling Safe

Feeling safe comes from the belief that you can do what is necessary to take care of yourself both physically and emotionally. It is a matter of trust. Through the process of assessment and reassurance, the belief that you can trust yourself to make decisions that are best for you begins to grow. You set boundaries for yourself and stand up for the values those boundaries represent. You look to your gut to tell you what feels comfortable for you and what doesn't. You remove yourself from situations and relationships that are physically or emotionally dangerous. You make the adjustments necessary to keep yourself feeling as comfortable as possible in situations and relationships that could be damaging, or that are simply less than perfect. You seek support for your decisions and help when you're confused, whether it's from friends, groups, or professionals.

You also give yourself the time and energy needed to maintain your positive feelings about what you are doing. Daily meditation books, regular breaks from your routine, doing something weekly just for yourself, plenty of sleep and rest, and engaging in a hobby and social situations are all ways to reinforce that you are worth the time and energy it takes to keep yourself in touch with the multi-faceted person you are. These are signs that you respect you and believe in yourself. This is the essence of self-worth.

Self-Worth

Self-worth is our motivation for maintaining our boundaries and self-care practices in the face of criticism, ridicule, or contrasting principles. It is a feeling of value and importance without conceit. When you truly believe in yourself and know your worth, you have no need to tell the world, because the world will see and know by your stance and your actions. Self-worth is private and personal. It is a "knowing" rather than a "believing."

Because you know you are worth being alive, that you are valuable in the world for no other reason than your individuality as a person adds something to the world that no one else can give it, you treasure yourself as something precious. You are also able to acknowledge the individuality of others, and know there is no better or worse, only different.

The higher your sense of self-worth, the easier it is for you to know your limits, respect them, and take steps to ensure that your surrounding environment and relationships are the best possible for you. It's this feeling of self-worth that allows you to feel empowered and self-confident, both of which are necessary to create and maintain the healthiest, happiest world for you and yours.

Feeling Empowered/Self-Confident

Feeling empowered comes from within. It is knowing in your gut that you are an adult capable of making responsible, mature decisions. It is a power that whispers rather than shouts, heard because of its intensity rather than its noise. You feel powerful enough not only to take care of business, but to ask for help when you need it. You feel powerful enough to not know everything, to not be able to do everything, and to prioritize according to what's healthiest for you.

Empowerment gives you the ability to make decisions while self-confidences gives you the ability to carry out those decisions. Self-confidence creates an attitude of being okay with who you are without making excuses for that, while knowing that adjustment and change are important when necessary. For example, I don't have to apologize for liking to laugh out loud, but I also know that some places or situations may not be an appropriate time to do so and I respect that.

Self-confidence is flexible without being wishy-washy. It allows you to try new things, knowing you may not like them all, and you are able to fail at something without feeling you are a failure. You are able to meet the challenges of life and accept the results as they may be, giving yourself a chance even when the odds are against you. You accept yourself for who you are, and walk through the world with your head held high. Self-confidence grants you permission to choose as you please and change your mind without blame or shame.

Making Choices/Acting on Decisions

Making personal choices that are healthiest is not always easy, but it is always important. You need to believe in yourself, possess that feeling of empowerment, and surround yourself with confidence in order to look at options, choose what works best for you in any given situation, and follow through on your decisions. Being an adult means you now have the power to makes the rules for yourself you once accepted without question from other adults in your life. It's a great responsibility, being an adult, but the rewards are just as great.

Eating the way you want, the way that's best for your body, means making choices and acting on decisions that others may not like or agree with. This is where the concept of self-care can be challenged by those who think they know what's best for you, or who want you to be someone who serves their purpose, not your own.

As the process of feeling safe within yourself, feeling your own sense of self-worth, feeling empowered as an adult, and having the self-confidence to be you evolves, carrying out your decisions becomes easier. Doing all this can be confusing or difficult and having a good support system for yourself will help make it all easier and less bewildering. You will make mistakes, second-guess yourself, or go against your old belief system at times, but it's all part of the process. As you practice, you will become more adept at listening to yourself and acting on what you hear from within rather than from without. The more you do this, the happier you will feel.

Happiness

The feeling of happiness is manifested within us when we consistently make choices that respect our own values and are in our own best physical and emotional interests. This doesn't mean we walk around with a silly grin on our face all the time, that we are inconsiderate of others, that we are selfish and unkind, or that we never have problems and their accompanying emotions. Rather, it means that we are, for the most part, genuinely pleased with our choices and decisions because we know we are taking care of ourselves to the best of our ability. We are staying as true to ourselves as possible, and feel less compromised in our gut. We basically like who we are and what we are doing, and it just feels good.

Being as it's not a perfect world, you may find yourself making choices that will have you feeling uncomfortable at times, but those will become fewer and farther between. You may find yourself challenged or confronted by someone who wants to hold you hostage emotionally; recognize it for what it is, and do what you have to until you can get to a safer place. As you continue to take care of yourself, you'll find yourself feeling better about who you are. Isn't that what happiness is all about?

Feeling Uncomfortable

There will be times when you find yourself making choices that leave you feeling uncomfortable. This is a part of life and relationships that can't always be helped. It's OK to be uncomfortable.

There are three main areas of life and relationships that cause us discomfort, although they may actually feel dangerous at the time. This is usually due to the fact that we haven't had a lot of practice in safe or healthy experiences with them. They are the areas in which we have often suffered much pain and damage, either through neglect, inappropriate care, or unhealthy examples by the adults in our childhood.

These three areas are –

1. **Emotions**
2. **Touch**
3. **Intimacy** (both physical and emotional)

While these three areas are the cornerstones of our existence as interactive social beings, they are also the areas in which we feel the most discomfort due to the threat they represent from our past. They are the areas where we feel the least able to cope and keep ourselves feeling safe. We have had a lot of practice denying or avoiding them by using food and eating behaviors to distract us from or try to bury our discomfort with them.

Emotions – emotions generate fear and discomfort because we haven't had enough practice acknowledging, accepting, and expressing our emotions appropriately. We've learned that certain emotions are OK, while others aren't. Sometimes we've learned to cover certain emotions with others that are more acceptable. For example, many men are taught that hurt, sad, confused, guilty, fear (in fact, most of their emotions) aren't allowed, and they cover them with anger. Many women are taught that anger isn't acceptable and cover it with sadness, tears, or false smiles and excuses. Much repressed anger appears as rage or depression. In essence, we've usually been taught to hide our feelings, and feel uncomfortable not only with our own, but with the feelings of others as well.

You've probably worked hard at denying or burying your emotions by reaching for food, not allowing yourself to eat, exercising or purging – any number of ways to distract yourself or run away from what you are feeling. As you begin to eat for your body's needs, you'll discover more emotions coming to the surface. Emotions are not to be feared, but welcomed. They let you know you're a living human being.

Rely on your support system to help you sort them out and become more comfortable with them. Notice them, acknowledge them, accept them. There are no right or wrong feelings, no good or bad emotions. We all have them, and to deny them is to deny a part of yourself.

One caution here – emotions can be connected to triggers of past events or situations where you were in danger if you expressed them. It's important to realize that getting in touch with emotions may need the help of a professional. This is an area where it's extremely important to go at your own pace, and with all the help you need.

The other part of having emotions is learning to express them appropriately. Tears are appropriate for sadness or pain; letting your anger out in a way that doesn't hurt you or anyone else is important; smiles and laughter express happiness and joy. Being comfortable with setting boundaries and choosing as you please helps dissolve guilt, and bringing shameful and fearful feelings into the light by talking about them extinguishes the shame and diminishes the fear.

Also, beware of "cousins." Irritation, sarcasm, habitual lateness, are all signs of repressed anger. Nervousness, worrying, anxiety are all related to fear. Excuses, verbal attacks, avoiding the subject reflect shame. These "cousins" send us to the refrigerator just as quickly as the identified major emotions.

Happiness and excitement, even though they're viewed as positive emotions, can also be uncomfortable enough to send us groping for something to put in our mouths. Emotions of any kind are stressful, and we've been taught to "quick-fix" stress instead of taking the time to look at it, acknowledge it, and do what's appropriate. We've been taught that when we do something positive, we deserve a treat. One of the best treats you can give yourself is at least one-half hour each day just to relax and make yourself a priority. It's probably one of the hardest things for you to do, but one of the most important.

Touch – the second area that causes us discomfort is touch. You may have experienced touch as painful, manipulative, threatening, or sexually unacceptable. These types of touch have crossed your personal boundaries in order to satisfy the rage, desires, or whims of another. The thought of someone touching you now can bring on great discomfort.

Touch is a human need, and to deny it will leave you feeling destitute within your very being. Those of us who haven't had very much touch in our lives are usually touch-deprived, and often trade sex, sports, or animals for healthy human touch. It has been shown that babies fail to thrive, and can die, when deprived of simple human touch. That very real situation occurred in England during World War II, when thousands of babies were sent out of London to avoid the bombings and there weren't enough adults to actually hold the babies, demonstrating this failure-to-thrive phenomenon.

Human beings need kind, caring, nonsexual touch several times a day. Babies and children provide the chance to touch another human being without fear. Pets are also popular for this reason: they provide their owners with touch that isn't regularly gotten from other humans. Pets are often used as the means to receive touch by people who feel threatened in some way by the touch of other adults, or who don't have adults in their lives to provide the touch they need.

Both men and women have had a lot of inappropriate sexual touch from both sexes, which not only distorts their own sexuality, but also their ways and means of giving and receiving sexual touch. Any hurtful touch that was somehow justified or denied by another (it's your fault, you made me do it, it was just a joke, don't be so sensitive, I was just playing, you deserved it, etc.) or not saying anything so that you had to guess at the reason for it, caused distortions in your sense of what touch can do and what it's used for.

Support groups and many therapist/counselors can provide a safe place to experience non-sexual, feel-good touch in the form of hugs. Therapeutic massage can also provide safe touch. It may take some getting used to, but you'll find that once your need for touch is being met in appropriate ways, food is no longer an adequate substitute.

Intimacy – there are two kinds of intimacy: physical and emotional. Physical intimacy is otherwise known as being sexual, while emotional intimacy is the act of feeling close to another even though there is no physical contact. Both carry a sense of vulnerability, the sense of being open to be hurt. It's this vulnerability that brings out the fear because of the idea that another person can use what you've shared against you. Even the threat or awareness of that can cause discomfort.

Healthy emotional intimacy means feeling cared about. Feelings are shared without the fear of ridicule, judgment, abuse, or being ignored, dismissed, or denied. Food has often been used to show love or care, either through its preparation, dining out, or even ordering a pizza. Any of these ways can be utilized to avoid talking about feelings. They can help you keep an emotional distance between the two of you.

Sexual intimacy means feeling cared about as well, in a physically pleasuring way. The focus is not just on receiving pleasure, but making sure your partner is feeling pleasured. Pleasure is shared without the fear of ridicule, judgment, abuse, or being ignored. Living up to expectations or fantasies about image or performance can cause extreme discomfort for either person. Food is often substituted as a way to stay connected while allowing the sexual side of the relationship to fade away. Using food to create a false sense of intimacy denies us of important aspects of a relationship and never fills the hollow feeling left by their absence.

Advertisers play on these fears by encouraging you to use food as a substitute for time, energy, caring, and sharing in relationships. They've told you that "lovin'" comes from what's in the oven, they've shown sensual images, usually with chocolate or ice cream, of licking, sucking, and sounds of pleasure, and they've encouraged the belief that the best way to show you care is by cooking for someone.

They reinforce many of the messages you may have gotten growing up. They encourage you to lose touch with your own personal messages, your own emotions, your own feelings, and your own natural responses to the situations you face each day. In reality, food presents an inadequate kind of substitute for being human and having healthy, caring, relationships with other humans.

The process of becoming familiar and comfortable with who you are on all levels takes time. Your goal is to learn how to eat according to the messages your body sends you. You've been eating in a non-natural manner for a long while. Allow yourself the time you need to realize more natural food selections and eating behaviors. This is for life.

Weekly Assignment

In order to get in touch with the fear behind your feelings of discomfort, the assignment is for you to keep a chart of the times you eat in order to comfort yourself while avoiding or feeling a lack in those three areas of touch, emotions, and intimacy. Do this for a week. The chart for Chapter IV is on Page (ix) of the Appendix. Fill in the date that you ate because you felt uncomfortable about something. Identify whether that discomfort was about an emotional issue, a touch issue, or an intimacy issue. Write down what kind of reassuring words that scared child within you would need to hear in order to dispel the fear and make you feel safer about that issue. Finally, write down some words of praise for yourself for having the courage to look at these issues, and for doing something positive for yourself.

For example, if you begin this chart on a Monday, write the dates for the entire week in the "Date" column. The first day you eat because of feeling uncomfortable about something, identify what's making you uncomfortable and write down in the "Emotions/Touch/Intimacy" column which area the discomfort was about.

In the "Reassurance" column, write some words that can reassure yourself you aren't in danger, you can deal with this situation appropriately, and you are able to keep yourself safe. Use whatever words work best for you. These are the missing words you've needed to hear during past situations of the same type. Give them to yourself now. See what they look like, how they feel to you, and how they make you feel about yourself.

Finally, in the "Praise" column, write some words of praise for yourself, words that give you a verbal pat on the back. Some examples might be "This was tough, but I did it," or "I'm not perfect at this, but I'm making progress," or even "Good for me."

This assignment is not designed to push you any farther that you are ready to go, but to give you an opportunity to begin looking at the issues that may be keeping you stuck in non-natural eating patterns. Ask for help if you need it, either from a professional, a trusted friend, or a support group. Use others to help you get to where you want to go at the speed most comfortable to you. Going too fast can be overwhelming, so take you time, and remember, you don't have to do this perfectly.

To Remember

- Addictions are about believing you can control something that has shown itself to be uncontrollable
- Elimination lets go of trying to control the uncontrollable
- Change is a process that takes time and patience
- You can give yourself the reassurance and comfort you need for your fears and pain
- For any situation in which you feel fear (nervousness, anxiety, worry, etc.), ask yourself if you're facing the lion or the roar
- Assessment is what allows you to distinguish between danger and discomfort.
- Danger can harm you, discomfort doesn't
- The "quick-fix" is appropriate for dangerous situations only
- It's OK to feel uncomfortable
- The three most uncomfortable areas are emotions, touch, and intimacy
- Food is not a substitute for caring about yourself other than nourishment

CHAPTER V

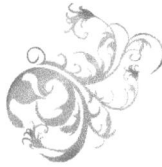

TAKING CONTROL

Assignment Review

Charting

The charts in this program can be used by you to gather information about your food choices, eating choices, and patterns. Whether you complete them or not is always up to you. They are simply provided as tools to help you sort out any confusion you may have about why, when, how, and what you eat in a self-destructive way.

The information collected from the charting exercises can also be used to more clearly understand the non-natural roles food and eating have played for you. By clarifying these roles for yourself, you will be more able to see how you have perceived food and eating as being something other than fuel for your body. This clarification helps you to see the specific areas which have developed into trouble spots for you and to design a different strategy for breaking your unhealthy cycles.

Chapter IV Chart

Turning now to the charting exercise for Chapter IV, you were asked to keep an account of the times you ate when you weren't hungry and to note from which one of the three areas of emotion, touch, or intimacy you were escaping or distracting yourself. This kind of information can help you become aware of some of the issues keeping you trapped in your self-destructive eating patterns.

What you are able to learn from this information is a recognition of some of the areas within the relationships you have with yourself and others that have an element of fear or the anticipation of pain about them. By beginning to identify these areas, you are taking steps to understanding the underlying reasons for the difficulty you've encountered in breaking your non-natural eating patterns. In essence, identifying these areas gives you insight into the nurturing role you have associated with food and eating.

The Chapter IV charting exercise allows you to begin understanding the idea that non-natural food perceptions and eating patterns have very little to do with food and eating. Instead, certain underlying issues, possibly beyond your conscious comprehension, have been directing not only your perceptions, but also your behaviors concerning food and its role in your life. It's in identifying these issues and bringing them into a conscious focus that allows you to begin to establish more realistic perceptions about food and healthier eating patterns.

Identifying the issue(s) or feelings that contribute to non-natural perceptions and patterns concerning food and eating may not automatically cause your behaviors to go away, but they will give you an idea of what is happening with you and why. These types of issues often have some deep underlying trauma or years of negative experience that have made them ingrained and often buried. Insights as to the nature of the underlying issues can in turn begin to suggest a different, more personally appropriate course of action for you to pursue.

One of these courses of action may include professional counseling or therapy, especially with someone who is familiar with eating issues and addictive processes. While you may have taken part in counseling in the past, this new focus can help you be more interactive regarding the direction any new counseling takes.

If at any time you start feeling overwhelmed or out of control because of issues that are revealed while you read this book, it's time to check in with a professional. Some of these issues, especially those concerning sexual abuse, chronic emotional abuse, repeated physical abuse, grief, and loss, may be more appropriate for a counseling session than talking with a friend or with a support group because of the depth of the issue and the intensity involved in its exploration. Individual counseling can help you get over a "hump" when you are stuck, and can give you the direction and tools for resolving these issues.

Unresolved issues that may be affecting your perception of food and eating include:

- death of a loved one or of a relationship (through divorce or separation)
- lack of a relationship with a significant other or unhappiness to any degree with a present relationship (feeling overwhelmed, unsatisfied, belittled, unimportant, smothered, distant, disrespected as an individual, or codependency by either partner, etc.)
- major transitions (births, deaths, children leaving home, marriage, job changes, moving, etc.)
- past trauma (sexual or physical abuse of any kind or intensity, witness to violence, any disruption of

your life or lifestyle when you had no power to change or prevent it, emotional or physical neglect, etc.)

- childhood and family issues (parents, siblings, stepparents, friends, relatives, neighborhood, lifestyle, etc.) that still interfere with present relationships and peace of mind
- any loss that you believed you had resolved but still affects you adversely
- self-esteem (only feeling good about yourself through your job, friends, being loved/liked, what you do, how much money you make, what your body looks like, how busy you are, how many problems you handle, how clean your house is, how well your children do, etc.)

These types of issues need to be addressed from an adult perspective with appropriate reassurance and comfort. It's through acknowledging your fear and feeling your pain that you will be able to resolve and leave these issues behind. This is often best done by talking with someone, professional or otherwise, to guide you and give you different, hopefully more realistic perceptions of the situation. It is never done by stuffing them away or distracting yourself with food and eating.

The Process of Change

Throughout the course of this program you have learned how your unconscious perceptions have a direct relationship to your sense of personal empowerment. Remember how drawing the perception of your body, and your emotions surrounding that perception gave you an idea of the unconscious negative personal environment you have been surrounding yourself with? Negativity on any level, whether conscious or unconscious, does not promote positive change. Instead, it keeps you from realizing your personal power.

Even if you believe on a conscious level you are able to do something, your unconscious belief will determine if you actually have that ability or not. Here is a demonstration for you to perform with a friend that illustrates this point: Have one person stand with an arm uplifted to shoulder height. This person, Person A, will attempt to hold their arm up while the other person, Person B, will attempt to push it down using only two fingers placed on the wrist.

For the first part of the demonstration, Person A will repeat to themselves "I can't hold my arm up." Repeat this sentence over and over. After several repetitions, Person B will place two fingers on the wrist of Person A and with gentle, but moderate pressure, attempt to lower the arm. For most people, the arm will lower without much trouble. It's important to note that this is **NOT** a test of strength or wills. It's a demonstration of the power of your subconscious.

Next, Person A will again hold up their arm and change one word in the sentence they repeat. Change "can't" to "can" so the sentence being repeated is "I can hold my arm up." Again, with gentle, but moderate pressure, Person B will attempt to lower the arm using only two fingers. Usually, Person A is able to maintain the arm at shoulder height without much difficulty, and person B would need to apply a much greater amount of pressure to push that arm down.

I have seen this demonstration work with both men and women, weight lifters and non-physically-fit people. The idea behind the demonstration is that there is power in your unconscious belief system. Your beliefs around the word "can't" are different, and actually power-sapping compared to those around the word "can." Even though you consciously wanted to hold that arm up, the beliefs at the unconscious level determined whether you truly had the power to do so.

This may be why you often *want* to do something, but find yourself seemingly unable to follow through. If your unconscious beliefs include statements about yourself of not being worth happiness, not being truly valuable as a person, or not being good enough to deserve love and kindness from yourself or anyone else, you will act in ways that support those beliefs. Consciously you may say you love yourself, but if your unconscious belief contradicts that, you will act in ways that contradict self-love. A person's behaviors are indicators of the true beliefs they have about themselves.

Through the Chapter III chart, you have recognized when and with what foods you are out of control. You have begun to identify situational patterns to non-natural eating choices. Through the Chapter IV chart, you are more familiar with how the various aspects of relationships, both with yourself and others, cause fear and the anticipation of pain in your life. You may also have begun to comprehend, in part, the scope of the self-perceptions that have triggered old, unhealthy, self-destructive behaviors.

These awarenesses can be extremely helpful in giving you an idea of what kinds of personal changes may be necessary in order to eat differently. They can also help you determine what your eating patterns are a substitute for, what may be missing from your life, and what it is you really want in your relationships.

Awareness doesn't automatically mean things will change, however. Another aspect needs to be considered when talking about change, and that is action. In other words, to make changes, you must be willing to take the risk of actually doing something new and different. This is what I call the "Double A" of change.

The process of changing food and eating patterns is much like learning to drive a stick-shift car. When you first learn, you need instruction and education in order to understand what driving with a stick-shift is all about. Driving stick usually seems complicated and confusing at first, especially when you are trying to remember which foot or which hand goes where.

Hearing the instructions more than once can help to clear up some of the confusion and straighten out the complexity of the process. Receiving encouragement and support for your efforts inspires you to continue when the going gets rough.

However, understanding will only take you so far. You won't learn how to do the actual driving until you get into the car and onto the road. It's through practice, trying out new concepts, making mistakes, learning from those mistakes, and repeating the process over and over that driving stick shift eventually happens. It's through taking the risk and *doing* what seemed nearly impossible in the beginning which allows you to change it into something that becomes nearly automatic on a day-to-day basis.

Changing your perceptions of food and eating and taking the steps necessary to eat differently are also a process. This program acts as the educational and instructional part of the process of change by giving you information and instruction on what to do to begin unravelling the complexity of it. Encouragement and support from others help you to stay focused on the behaviors you want to change. Just like with driving a stick-shift, you are the only one who can actually do what's necessary to get your own process moving.

It's important to realize, however, that even though this process may become quite automatic for you over time, it doesn't mean you will ever be perfect at it. I've been driving stick shift for over 50 years and I still occasionally grind the gears, stall the car, or roll backwards down a hill. The difference between coping with those mistakes now and in the past is that now I have a much quicker response to the situation, and am able to recover faster and more efficiently. The goal to strive for is consistency. Be gentle with yourself when you "grind the gears." We all do it once in a while.

What Food and Eating Mean to You

Because food and eating have not always meant very much in the way of fueling your body, they must have other meanings for you. These meanings can run the gamut from showing how in control you are to how out of control you are, what a friend you have in food, or how distracting food and eating can be when you are faced with an uncomfortable situation. The surface meanings for food choices and eating patterns may be different for everyone, but underneath they all serve the same function -- they have given you a false sense of power in situations where you feel powerless.

The idea of feeling powerless means you have probably reverted to an emotional state of being a child. It's in childhood where you didn't have much power over situations that caused you fear and pain. You didn't have a lot of choices except to put up with the situation in any way possible in order to survive it with your body and mind reasonably intact.

Trying to control too much fear and pain can seem overwhelming to a child in a very real sense. It's when attempting to deal with, manage, or handle such large amounts of fear and pain that the child looks for whatever can help to control the feeling of being overwhelmed. In attempting to take control of that which feels out of control, food choices and eating patterns are given their power. In order to survive some very ugly, frightening, and often life-threatening situations, you did whatever was necessary to make it through alive, both physically and emotionally.

The concept of "life-threatening" can take on different meanings for different situations with different people. There are the obvious physical threats and fears, but there are also the more devious emotional threats and fears. Even though many people believe they can take care of themselves physically, they may not feel so sure about taking care of themselves emotionally. This feeling of emotional vulnerability can feel life-threatening.

Being in touch with your feelings, being able to express them appropriately, being comfortable with nurturing touch, and allowing yourself intimacy in your relationships are all concepts that can feel life-threatening to an individual. Using food and eating as a substitute or distraction may start at any time in your life as a way to cope or as a means to emotional survival.

The child has few resources for coping appropriately with anything that seems overwhelming and is, therefore, quite powerless to effect any significant change in an appropriate manner. Without the help of adults, the child must use childish coping strategies. While these may be effective for a while, as the child grows without learning and practicing more mature responses and reactions, the strategies become less effective. Eventually, the adult is attempting to cope with uncomfortable situations from the same perspective as a child, using similar, childish strategies, and feeling as powerless as a child to bring about appropriate change.

The belief that something feels life-threatening to you as an adult revolves around the belief that you don't have the power to cope with a situation in a way that will keep you feeling safe and able to deal with the pain. As a child, you very often didn't have the power to change a situation or remove yourself from the people who were hurting you. This powerless feeling was often terrifying, yet it was something you had to cope with in any way possible. One of the ways to cope with it may have been through food and eating.

In a sense, then, food choices and eating patterns have seemed like lifesavers in situations that felt dangerous and in which you felt out of control and powerless. This is the reason it has been so difficult to change these patterns and choices. Without gaining new, more powerful coping skills for whatever situation in which you feel fear or anticipate pain, you revert to what has helped you survive in the past.

Learning about your own personal fear "triggers" helps you to understand more about the situations in which you feel powerless. As explained in Chapter IV, three major areas for producing fear in people are the areas of emotions, touch, and intimacy. These are the areas in which most people feel powerless and out of control. The combination of these two feelings produce fear and the anticipation of pain. Eating patterns and food choices then play their parts as reassurance and comfort agents.

Through the first two charting exercises you have become aware of how often you turn to food during times of fear and pain. These are the times you have felt incapable of coping with a situation in a way that would keep you reassured and feeling safe. Because you feel as powerless as a child, you revert to using one of the behaviors that has given you the perception of power and control and has meant reassurance and comfort for you throughout your life.

The Child Within

The times you use eating/not eating *as* an adult to take the place of the reassurance and/or comfort you need are very similar to the times you looked *to* an adult for reassurance and comfort as a child. At these times in your childhood you felt afraid and wanted an adult to take care of you and fix the situation. You wanted an adult to reassure you that you were safe and everything would be all right. You wanted someone to be powerful and in control of the situation for you.

I believe if we didn't get what we needed from adults when we were children, we get stuck at that particular place of perception and continue into adulthood with similar childhood perceptions and fears. If these childhood issues aren't resolved in an appropriate manner, we stay emotionally stuck at that stage and attempt to resolve other such conflicts when we become adults as we would have at that particular emotional developmental time in childhood.

Relating this concept of development to comfort and reassurance, when we were afraid as children and were unable to get the reassurance we needed from the adults we depended on to take care of us, we became stuck in that child place of fear. When we were hurt, either physically or emotionally, and were unable to get the comfort we needed, we became stuck in that child place of pain. Being stuck there has meant that we continue into our own adulthood not knowing how to give ourselves the reassurance and comfort we need when we anticipate a situation to be dangerous and/or painful.

In other words, you become an adult without the knowledge or skills you have needed in order to give that child within you the reassurance and comfort that child needs for being afraid or in pain. The result is that as an adult you feel afraid, and it is often the child part of you which is perceiving some danger. When you are in pain, you feel overwhelmed, as a child might be, with the idea of being vulnerable. You become stuck in that place of fear and pain because the adult part of you doesn't know how to give reassurance and comfort to yourself. You revert to feeling the situation is somehow life-threatening, and that you won't be able to survive it.

Not only do you feel unable to keep yourself safe but you don't believe you are able to cope with the situation or problem at hand in an appropriate manner. Along with fear and pain, you have been stuck at a child's level of comprehension and perception of your own sense of power. The ability to both recognize the source of your discomfort so you are able to move from the child's level to the adult's level of assessment, perception, and power has been missing.

Child-Adult Perspectives

There is a vast difference between a child's perspective and the perspective of an adult when it comes to situation response and problem resolution. Children view and experience things with fewer options and less power for coping with them. When you are stuck at a child's level of perception and feelings, you believe you have few options, and very limited power to implement those options. This difference is what gets in the way of consistently coping appropriately with situations and problems as an adult.

That's not to say we don't accomplish many adult tasks in our lives-- we drive cars, we vote, we hold jobs, we raise children--but often when we are confronted with certain situations or problems, we don't know if we have the ability to cope with the consequences of adult decisions and choices. We get stuck in a child's place of not knowing how to handle the situation or resolve the problem appropriately, and we end up feeling nervous, anxious, and ultimately afraid we will be failures and that the pain of being a failure will be overwhelming.

It is this fear that needs to be addressed and assessed from an adult perspective. When it isn't, you are prevented from coping with situations and problems in an adult manner. Reverting to that child perspective within yourself is not bad or wrong, but remaining there keeps you trapped in self-destructive cycles. Moving out of it into a more adult perspective is what allows you to take action in a more adult manner, and enables you to accomplish whatever it is you truly want to do.

Child-Adult Problem Solving

In order to make such an assessment and move yourself into a more adult perspective of the situation or problem at hand, it's important to know where you are stuck. The chart on Page (x) of the Appendix gives you an overall view of how the perspectives of children and adults differ when faced with a problem to solve.

On the chart, there are six categories containing both a child's perspective and an adult's perspective of each particular area. Both these perspectives will be explained, along with the consequences for holding onto a child's perspective as an adult. It is important to note that for a child, a child's perspective is appropriate. It is simply part of being a child. For an adult, however, remaining within a child's perspective encourages unhealthy behaviors and relationships. This includes your relationship with food and eating.

Dependency-Survival Ability/Capability

Child's Perspective -- Children are dependent on others for their very existence. Children need someone to take care of them, to provide for their basic needs of food, shelter, clothing, and medical attention or they will die. Children also depend on adults to buffer them from the rest of the world. They rely on adults for their emotional well-being and to define the way they view themselves. They depend on adults to keep them safe in order for them to survive physically, emotionally, mentally, and spiritually.

Adult with a Child's Perspective -- When adults look at the world from a child's perspective in this area, they may become co-dependent with others and often have problems with feelings of abandonment and rejection if a relationship doesn't go the way they want it to go. They usually attempt to maintain relationships with very little sense of autonomy and independence for either partner. Change in the relationship or by the partner is seen as threatening because of the fear of being left behind. These adults often stay in destructive, abusive relationships because they feel safer in a relationship they know and understand (no matter how much it hurts them) rather than being on their own in the world. Their belief in being able to stand up for or take care of themselves independently is often non-existent.

Adult Perspective -- Adults with an adult perspective concerning their dependency/survival abilities/capabilities are consistently inter-independent. That is, they know both that they can survive on their own and be happy, but that they are intrinsically social creatures and need other caring people around them in order to flourish. These adults realize people come and go from their lives, and are not afraid to leave old, unhealthy relationships behind. They believe they will do what it takes to provide for themselves in a healthy manner and take care of themselves no matter who is or isn't a part of their lives.

Knowledge/Experience Base

Child Perspective -- Children operate in a very small space when it comes to knowledge and experience. By virtue of the fact that they just don't have a lot of life time behind them, they don't have a lot of living to draw from for examples and options. Children often believe in magical solutions to problems and spend a lot of their time in fantasy. Much of their experience includes extremely limited ways of looking at the world and they usually function within an "all or nothing" arena.

Adult with a Child's Perspective -- Adults looking at the world with a child's perspective continue to see the resolution of many situations and problems in an "all or nothing" manner. They usually believe they only have either/or options and often feel trapped between the proverbial rock and a hard place. They see their options as being exceedingly limited and may consistently exhibit behaviors of one extreme or another. These adults often experience a lot of fear and the feeling of being out of control in their lives, but may express such feelings as a lot of unresolved anger at their limited circumstances. Reality is very difficult to deal with when these adults often remain stuck trying to "wish" their way out of feeling trapped, as in "if only I won the lottery, I wouldn't have any more problems."

Adult Perspective -- Adults with an adult perspective toward their knowledge and experience base make choices based on the reality of the situation, knowing that the way they see something isn't necessarily the only way to look at it. These adults consider a situation from many angles in order to broaden the base of their perspective as much as is achievable in the time available. If they can't find a workable solution on their own, they ask for options and opinions from other people. They work to find the gray areas of resolution to their problems and rarely engage in extreme behaviors.

Time/Comprehension

Child Perspective -- Children have very little sense of actual time, and they lack the comprehension to understand the concept of time. For them, ten minutes can seem as long as ten hours. For this reason, children are demanding and believe in "now or never." They entertain a "quick-fix" mentality, often feeling panicky and in danger when an uncomfortable situation or problem isn't resolved immediately. They don't know they can take the time to resolve a problematic situation in an appropriate way, and that they will survive during the time it takes to do so.

Adult with a Child's Perspective -- Adults who have a child's perspective of time and comprehension retain a "quick-fix" mentality of needing to find solutions to situations and problems RIGHT NOW! These adults have difficulty taking the time needed for realistic assessment of a situation and lack the patience to take the time needed for appropriate resolution. They are usually rushed, try to do many things at once, and often wind up doing too much and suffering from burnout and/or physical and emotional exhaustion. They also have a difficult time with the idea of making mistakes and often feel panicky at the prospect of being less than perfect. They often experience a lot of fear of not getting everything done "on time."

Adult Perspective -- The adults with an adult perspective are patient rather than panicky. They know that they can take the time needed to explore the situation or problem in order to make conscious adult decisions about the best way to cope. Realistic time elements are understood, and, except in the case of an emergency, these adults know that things don't have to be fixed "right now." Their assessment is done in an individual time frame, one that tolerates their personal capacity and competence for coping in the given situation or with the specific problem.

These adults also know that if they aren't able to cope with the problem alone, there is usually help available in the form of feedback, opinions, and options which can be gathered from various other sources, including friends, family, ministers, support groups, and other professionals. In this way these adults relegate the feelings of fear and danger to more manageable levels of discomfort and caution. The fear ceases to be overwhelming and they cope with the situation or problem in a more appropriate manner.

Focus/Individuation

Child Perspective -- Children's sense of who they are is fragile, and because of this, children depend on first, the opinions of adults (believing everything they say and imply about the child, whether it's true or not) and second, how they compare to others (especially in adolescence) in order to get a working representation of not only what they are actually like but what they *should* be like. This focus on others can impede them from being able to stick to their own opinions if there is a conflict, and conflict resolution may be accomplished by denying the self. For children, their sense of self exists through the eyes of others, and their focus stays on others as a means to knowing about themselves.

Adult with a Child's Perspective -- Adults who remain in the child's perspective of focus and individuation continue to be focused on others for their sense of self. They constantly compare themselves to others, either in real life, from books, or through the media, in order to get a sense of what they *should* be or look like. They spend a lot of time, energy, and money trying to mold themselves to someone else's idea of "right" while denying their own individuality.

When they don't live up to these outside expectations, they believe something is wrong with them, never realizing the outside messages could be what's wrong. These adults continue to work at living up to unrealistic standards, believing all the opinions and feedback they receive as ultimate truth, which causes them to never be satisfied with who they are or what they look like. They are in a constant searching mode, always striving to improve themselves against some outside judgment.

Adult Perspective -- Adults with an adult perspective about where their focus needs to be and their own sense of individuation accept that they are not perfect, never will be, and stop trying to attain perfection. Instead, these adults look at themselves realistically, accept themselves for the flawed but wondrous creatures they are, and continue to move in a direction that capitalizes on their strengths while diminishing their weaknesses.

These adults are also realistic about what these strengths and weaknesses are and eliminate absolutes (such as believing only the best, strongest, prettiest, are good enough, etc. or believing no one could like someone so ugly, dumb, clumsy, etc.). They keep the focus on themselves as the foremost authority for what fits or what works best in their lives. They listen to and trust the messages from their inner selves. These adults may seek affirmation from others for these messages, but they ultimately trust their own messages as the ones to believe and act on. They know they are OK, no better and no worse than any other human being, singularly individual yet a valuable part of humankind.

Self-Worth/Self-Value

Child Perspective -- Children intrinsically have a solid sense of their self-worth and value when they are born. However, due to their dependence on adults, they may receive an altered sense of what they're worth from the messages provided them by those adults who are most responsible for their care and well-being. Children accept as a fact that adults know more than they do about themselves, and believe the opinions and judgments pronounced upon them, whether these opinions and judgments agree with their own original sense of worth and value or not.

Based on messages they get from others, including how much time and energy they are given by the people most important in their lives, they may alter their own sense of worth and value. They question how much they matter to those around them and to the world as a whole.

Adult with a Child's Perspective -- Adults who look at the world with the perspective of a child retain as true much of everything anyone has ever said about them and often live their lives at the one extreme of trying to prove it or at the other extreme of trying to disprove it. Along with spoken messages, they also retain messages implied by expectations, body language, and reactions to them by the adults around them.

These adults don't have a strong sense of their own worth and value in the world, often believing it's everyone else who deserves the good stuff, and that they themselves are lucky to get any bits and pieces that might be left over. These adults don't have a strong investment in themselves because they don't believe they're worth it. They allow others to determine what's OK for them and often settle for what comes their way without believing they're worth the energy of asserting themselves to strive for what they truly want.

Adult Perspective -- Adults who view the world with an adult perspective about their worth and value have a strong sense of knowing the fact that they exist makes a difference in the world. They believe in the idea that they deserve the best, and aren't ready to settle for less if they can help it, including the way they are treated in their relationships, the kinds of work they do, and the care they give themselves.

They expect to be treated with respect, and they show others by example how they respect themselves. These adults have a personal investment in themselves that enables them to make time for their own needs while being considerate of the needs of others. Their outlook is generally optimistic and they have faith that they can cope with situations and problems as they come along.

Personal Empowerment

Child's Perspective -- Children, by the very nature of their status in our society, have little power, either to make changes in their lives or to enforce their personal boundaries. They are regulated by the rules and boundaries of the adults in charge of them, whether those rules and boundaries are totally controlled by the adults at one extreme, or are totally left to the children to determine at the other extreme.

Children must live at the whim of adults, and depending upon how the adults handle these rules and boundary-holding processes, they can have responsibility withheld or thrust upon them at inappropriate ages and for inappropriate reasons. They don't have a lot of responsibility for the direction their lives take and they usually don't have a lot to say about it, either. They are easily victimized through the fact that they are naive, inexperienced, and without the capability to understand adult motivation.

Adult with a Child's Perspective -- Adults looking at their lives with the perspective of a child continue to feel powerless, even though they may have as much power as anyone else to determine the course of their lives. They remain in a victim role in their relationships, complaining about how they are mistreated, used, and abused, or they become victimizers of others, following the examples of what had been done to them.

Adults with very little sense of personal empowerment often live in extremes. They either look to others for advice on every decision facing them, or they scorn advice of any kind. They let others intimidate them or they intimidate others.

These adults either allow people to take advantage of them through a passive sense of not asserting their own personal boundaries, often because they don't realize they have a right to determine those boundaries, or they are aggressive in their boundaries, inconsiderate of the boundaries of others in order to get what they want or what they believe they deserve to have.

Adult Perspective -- Adults with an adult perspective about personal empowerment know this type of power comes from within themselves, and it doesn't have to be displayed or shown off to be felt and utilized. These adults take responsibility for their actions, determining which of their own personal choices have resulted in their present situation, and learning from any mistakes they might make. They own their part in any interaction. While they look for opinions and feedback when faced with important situations and decisions in their lives, they sift through the information they gather and ultimately make up their own minds. They determine not only what they want from their lives, but also what kinds of people they themselves want to be, and take the appropriate actions to correspond with their choices.

These adults have a strong sense of what is and isn't OK for them, and they set up and respectfully enforce their personal boundaries. They are strong yet gentle, caring about others yet they take care of themselves, and they are confident that whatever comes along in their lives, they can cope.

Bridging the Gap

There is a gap between these two perspectives that needs to be bridged in order to move from a child's perspective to an adult's perspective. The difference in these perspectives means the difference in dealing with situations and problems in a healthy, adult way, or an unhealthy, inappropriate way. Continuing in your life as an adult operating through a child perspective means either dealing with problems, situations, and conflicts in a way that consistently tries to please others and denies yourself, or that has no regard for others whatsoever and denies their rights and boundaries. Either you end up feeling used, abused, and cheated out of something that is rightfully yours, or you attempt to abuse and cheat others out of what is rightfully theirs.

This gap is filled with pain and fear, which is what keeps us from being able to move from a child's perspective to an adult's perspective. By remaining on the child side of the gap, the ability to perceive and thereby deal with problematic situations in an adult manner is denied you. When such situations arise, the fear and anticipation of pain rear their ugly heads and, instead of confronting them, and walking through them, you attempt to bury them or distract yourself from them by using food and eating.

In essence, you keep yourself from reaching an adult perspective and way of dealing with situations because food and eating are used as the fillers for this gap. Unfortunately, they are insubstantial for such a task. They aren't appropriate for the pain and fear that lay within the gap, and, therefore, they give way when you attempt to use them for support. You end up with the same gap between where you are and where you want to be.

This is why it's so difficult to do what you actually want to do. This is why you feel trapped. This is why, after dieting and losing weight, you regain all your weight and more. You haven't learned what you need to know to bridge that gap and see things from an adult perspective. Therefore, you haven't been able to take action in an adult manner and you remain viewing and handling problematic situations as a child would.

Because that gap contains your fears and the threat of pain, the only things that will allow you to cross over to an adult perspective is to fill the gap with what truly belongs there. You need to address that fear and pain with what is appropriate for fear and pain. Food and eating are appropriate for hunger and nourishment. Reassurance and comfort are what are appropriate for fear and pain.

Reassuring and Comforting Yourself

Bridging the gap appropriately means acknowledging what is truly there, confronting it, and walking through the frightening roar. Something different must be done than what you've tried in the past. You look at the reality before you and make a realistic choice. In essence, it means that you decide what you want to do from an adult perspective.

It does *not* mean that you can never go back. You will always have the choice to return to your old ways of resolving problematic situations. In fact, depending on circumstances, sometimes you may want to. Sometimes you may just try your old ways of eating because it seems quicker and easier. However, the more you face your fears and pain, the less you will feel the need to go back and rely on food and eating as the means to reassure and comfort yourself.

In the previous chapter, the concepts of reassurance for fear and comfort for pain were discussed, and three major areas that produce fear and pain were addressed. The charting exercises have given you an idea about what food and eating have meant for you and where you have consistently been using food or eating as a way to prevent the fear and pain from overwhelming you. This chapter presented you with information about how a child perspective can take precedence over an adult perspective and how it ineptly attempts to deal with any situation in your life that presents the threat of fear and pain.

This knowledge now gives you quite a comprehensive idea of the role food and eating have played in your life and why. By using this new-found understanding, you may now be able to pinpoint most of the areas that are troublesome for you. You may now begin to identify your fears, understand where they might be coming from, and initiate the assessment needed to determine if there is actual danger present or if it is merely an uncomfortable situation.

It is not expected that you do this on your own. You may need help, because these fears are often long-standing and the pain associated with them can feel overwhelming. It is at this point that professional help may give you the support and encouragement you need to look at, acknowledge, and face your fears.

These fears are very real, and to try to trivialize them would be a mistake. However, there is a reason for these fears that usually originated in another time, in another place, in a different situation, and with different people. The reality of this could be the beginning of the reassurance you need to know that they may no longer represent a danger to you. If there is still a real danger present, it could suggest that you may eventually, and as quickly as possible, want to get out of such a dangerous situation.

Realizing some of your fears no longer hold the power over you they once had can be a beginning for you to bridge the gap between the child perspective and the adult perspective. To bridge the gap completely means to render the fears ineffective and to feel and survive the anticipated pain. It means you confront your fear and give yourself the reassurance you need that everything will be all right, that you will not be damaged beyond repair, and that you will not die. It means you feel the pain, give yourself the comforting words and actions appropriate to the situation, and realize the pain will eventually diminish. Even though there might be a scar, you will heal and go on with your life.

In order to give yourself the reassurance and comfort you truly need, it is imperative you acknowledge the adult part of you. While there are undoubtedly times when you are looking at situations from a child perspective, there are also undoubtedly times when you look at situations from an adult perspective. At these times you deal with problems, conflicts, and other types of situations in an adult manner, feel satisfied with the results, or learn from the mistakes.

It is this adult side of you that needs to be present for the child side of you when you are feeling trapped, afraid, and unable to appropriately deal with a situation. As you learn more about yourself and what your child side fears, you will have the capacity to begin giving yourself the reassurance and comfort you truly need from your adult side.

The underlying dynamic here is that the child part of you is looking for an adult to take care of everything. Your emotional child is looking to an adult, much like you did when you were actually a child, to assess the situation, reassure you that you will be OK, and provide comfort through words and action to let you know you will survive the pain intact.

Bridging the gap is a five-step process:

1 -- **Recognize**
2 -- **Assess**
3 -- **Reassure**
4 -- **Comfort**
5 -- **Review**

1 -- *Recognize that you are afraid.* Admit and accept your fear. You may not always be able to pinpoint exactly what it is you are afraid of, but a big first step is to acknowledge you are afraid, and that it's OK to be afraid.

2 -- *Assess the situation.* Realistically look for its danger potential. You may need help with this. It's OK to get opinions and feedback from others. After all, you have been acting from a perspective of danger for so long, it may be difficult to get a true reading on a situation for a while. Depending on whether the situation holds true danger or is merely one of discomfort, you will now be able to either begin to eliminate the situation or allow it to just "be."

3 -- *Reassure yourself for your fear.* If you are truly in a dangerous situation, you need to know you will do what needs to be done in order to get out of it. This may take time, and it may be a process, but it's reassuring to know an adult will take care of that scared child within.

If your situation isn't dangerous, but only uncomfortable, *you need to know you are able to cope with it,* either on your own or with help. The reassurance you give yourself is that whatever is going on, you will get through it, it won't last forever, and you will survive. You reassure yourself that your fear, while real, is not something to actually be afraid of.

4 -- *Comfort yourself.* Comforting yourself is similar to reassuring yourself. It's important to talk to yourself and say the words you need to hear to know this pain won't last forever, and that you will survive it. Give yourself a hug. Do what it is you need to have done to feel cared about and worth the time and energy it takes to be comforted.

5 -- *Review the situation.* Look at what's going on from an adult perspective and make choices appropriate for the situation. Feel your empowerment as an adult. Know you are worth taking care of. Get feedback and opinions from others. Make an adult decision.

As you practice these steps, not only will they become easier, but they will contribute to a healthier, more positive personal environment to surround yourself with. Your feeling of safety will increase, your self-confidence and sense of personal empowerment will expand, and you will be able to more consistently make choices and carry out actions that are truly beneficial and satisfactory for your life.

In the end, your overall sense of happiness will intensify. You will do more of the things you want to do, things that you like, and things which enhance your life. In the meantime, you will be eating more appropriately both the foods and amounts your body requires.

This process does not come about overnight, nor is it necessarily smooth. You will have starts and stops, you will stumble and slip, and sometimes you will even think you have gone backwards, perhaps all the way back to square one. Don't be discouraged. Hang on. This process takes time and energy. Every day is a new day. Every mistake can be learned from. There is no right way to do it, only the way that ultimately works best for you.

As you become more familiar with your own different areas of child and adult perspectives, you will have a better idea of where you've been trapped and where you want to go. If you find you remain trapped in a child perspective and can't seem to find the reassurance and comfort for yourself to enable you to bridge the gap, you may be looking at an area where professional help would be appropriate.

Assignment

The assignment for this chapter, and for the following week, is one last chart—Page (xi) of the Appendix. This chart will help you to determine where you get stuck in a child perspective. On a daily basis, watch for problems or situations for which you use food or eating as a coping mechanism. During the week, write these problems and situations down, what food or eating choices you used to cope with each, and what would be a more appropriate way of coping. Make a note for yourself as to what type of reassurance you would need to help make the transition from a child's "quick-fix" perspective to an adult's problem-solving perspective.

If you feel able to and OK about it, you might begin giving yourself the actual reassurance and comfort you need for some of the less threatening situations you find yourself in. Don't expect perfection. This is an opportunity to begin taking back control. It's also an opportunity to learn about yourself, what is best for you, what works, and what doesn't work.

This charting exercise is just another tool that can help you to discover what has been missing, what has helped keep you trapped in a self-destructive cycle of food and eating, and how to begin climbing out of the bottomless pit of feeling out of control. It won't happen overnight, but with perseverance, patience, and the knowledge that there is hope, you will start taking control and break the destructive cycles in which you have been trapped.

To Remember

- The more you know about yourself, the easier it is to determine what has been missing and what you need to add

- Courage comes from acknowledging fear, and strength is shown by the ability to be vulnerable.

- Our conscious actions belie our unconscious beliefs about ourselves

- Food and eating have provided *perceived* protection during *perceived* life-threatening situations and problems

- Using food and eating inappropriately takes away personal power

- Remaining within a child perspective continues self-destructive cycles

- To bridge the gap from a child perspective to an adult perspective means to risk doing something new and different

- Reassurance and comfort are appropriate responses to fear and pain

- You can provide reassurance and comfort for yourself by yourself, by calling a supportive friend, by seeking professional help, or by utilizing any number of relaxation or spiritual methods. You can also use a combination of these.

- Moving yourself to a more adult perspective is a process. It takes time and energy. The more you practice, the easier it will become.

CHAPTER VI

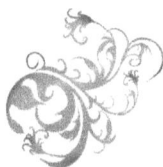

FEARS AND SABOTAGE

Assignment Review

Chapter V Chart

Before you explore this final chapter and learn about the ways in which you may not only fear success but also often sabotage your progress, let's review the charting exercise from Chapter V. This chart was designed to help you break your "automatic" eating response by encouraging you to think from an adult perspective and acknowledge the more appropriate responses to a situation or problem.

For example, let's say that one situation you charted during the week had to do with listening to your mother criticizing your weight. In the past you may have dealt with such criticism by rebelling (eating more than you were hungry for in an attempt to "show" her you can do what you want), feeling hurt (since she doesn't approve of you no matter how many other accomplishments you have under your belt, you eat to cover up the pain), or getting angry (and eating instead of letting her know how you feel). These are often responses from your "child" perspective.

This time, however, you decide you want to respond from an adult perspective. In doing so, you will progress through a number of stages of personal awareness, including:

- acknowledging your fear of not having your mother's approval, and your anger at her for butting into your business and treating you like a child.

- comforting that child part of you by letting it know it's OK to be afraid, and reassuring that frightened child part of you that the adult part of you will take care of the situation.

- understanding there's no real danger, and the fear doesn't have to stop you from doing what's healthiest for you anymore. (Here's where you bridge the gap between the child perspective and the adult perspective).

- acknowledging to yourself that you are an adult now and you do have the power to eat and weigh what you want, and you don't have to use food or your weight as a way to "show" your mom you have control of your life.

- thanking your mom for her input and/or telling her how you're feeling about it. This response often ends the conversation in its tracks. If not, you might mention something along the lines that you're working on it and you're sensitive about it, and you'd love it if she would support you in your effort.

Talking to your mother in an adult way helps to get you out of the parent-child communication pattern and into a more adult-adult type of relationship. Responding to feedback from an adult perspective is important no matter who is giving the feedback. The important thing to remember is that you don't need to argue about what she may or may not be doing – it may feel like criticism to you, but to her it may simply be motherly advice. It might just be better for you at this point to reiterate that this is a sensitive subject for you right now and you'd rather talk about something else for a while. It's not up to you to try to prove a point with her. She knows what she's doing and you can let it go.

Another charting example might have to do with having an argument with your partner or spouse. Dealing with this situation from a child perspective might include giving in, having a tantrum, or being dishonest about your feelings. You don't tell your partner what this situation means to you or how you feel about the whole thing. You end up at the refrigerator or cookie jar, or starving yourself for a few more days, or running to the gym for a few hours, frantically trying to work off your frustration and anger.

Responding from an adult perspective might include the following:

- Taking some time out in order to think about and acknowledge what you're feeling.
- Acknowledging the fear your child self feels for not being good enough to stand up for yourself or the possibility you will be rejected or abandoned because of your opinion.
- Reassuring your child within that you will cope with whatever happens, that you deserve to be who you are in this relationship, and that you have a right to be angry if that's how you feel.
- Comforting that child within by letting them know this relationship with yourself is worth some pain, that it won't

kill you, and above all it's important for you to be true to yourself (bridging the gap between child and adult perspective).

- Acknowledging the adult part of you that knows you have power to take care of yourself and give that part permission to act as a powerful adult.

- Return to your partner, use "I" statements to tell them how you feel and your viewpoint about the situation. Ask if there's any way the two of you can look for other options for settling the disagreement, if you can sit down and both present your own perspectives on the situation, or what else the two of you can do to reach an agreement.

- Feel the intimacy building and know that as an adult, this is what you really want instead of distracting yourself or burying your emotions through the use of food and eating.

While your own individual scenario might not proceed exactly like these examples, they give you an idea of some of the steps to take and some of the responses that are possible to make when striving to bridge the gap between the child and adult perspective. The main objective is to acknowledge both your child and adult sides so that you can reassure and comfort the child while feeling and utilizing the power of the adult. There are no contests to win. There is only the opportunity to be true to yourself as a whole human being.

This charting exercise is something you can use for the rest of your life when you feel trapped in a situation. It will give you time to slow down and figure out what is actually going on with you and what you really want to do about it. It is a tool to utilize anytime you feel you're uncomfortable in a situation. Although it may feel awkward in the beginning, the more you get to know yourself, the quicker and easier it becomes.

The Total You

Learning about and understanding yourself is a lifetime commitment. The more you learn and understand who you are and what you want, the easier it becomes to make those tough decisions you will face during the course of your life. Becoming aware of and acknowledging all the different parts of you makes it less difficult to bridge the gap between the child and adult perspective. In turn, your choices and behaviors continually become more adult-oriented, your life becomes more personally satisfying, and in the process, you are able to relegate food and eating to their proper places.

Looking at the total you can be frightening. There are probably things about yourself you've been running away from or attempting to bury for many years. This fear of admitting to and acknowledging who you really are can be stressful at times: you might feel anger, shame, and/or sadness, and these emotions might be painful.

That's why so many people avoid them for so long. We have all done things we're not especially proud of. Usually it's because that's how we protected or defended ourselves from the untruths we were told about what kind of person we are. Those were the means we had to survive, and it's important to know that you can start doing things differently now.

It's OK to forgive yourself for past behaviors and move on. It can be frightening to look at yourself this closely, and it may mean accepting some imperfect parts of you, which can also be painful. Unfortunately, there is no other way to bridge that gap than to face those fears and be ready and willing to make it through the pain.

Getting to know the total you may also be energizing and exhilarating. You will discover unknown strengths and talents, and possibly new ways to put them to use in your life. You can explore the different emotions you encounter about both positive and negative situations. You can also clarify your own perspective and more easily decide about choices and options. This provides the feeling of being more grounded and solid in who you are.

Learning more about yourself and what makes you tick allows you to examine what kind of person you are, not as a way to feel guilty about what you're not doing right, but as a way to decide what you want to keep and what you want to change. In the end, you will find you are like everyone else – a naturally flawed yet gloriously unique human being with your own individual way of seeing and reacting to the world. We all have strengths and weaknesses. None of us are perfect. We make mistakes. You don't have to be afraid of being who you are anymore.

Fears

Part of learning about yourself as a total human being includes discovering where your fears are when it comes to maintaining the positive steps you have already taken. Many people talk about starting something new and different that they like, that feels good, or that is good for them, but not continuing with it for very long, and actually going back to old, unhealthy behaviors. They don't understand why they do this, and often become frustrated to the point where they become resigned to never changing. They believe something is wrong with them and put themselves down, adding self-hate to their negative personal environment.

If you are one of these people, know that there is nothing wrong with you. However, there may be an undiscovered fear working at a sub-conscious level. This fear (there may even be more than one) could be preventing you from continuing down the path of self-care. It's not until you realize it's there, acknowledge its presence, and identify what it means that you will be able to face your fear and become powerful enough to walk through it.

Several fears have a common thread when it comes to breaking bad habits, changing self-destructive behaviors or recovering from addictions. The following examples may or may not be yours, but they might give you an idea of what to look for in yourself when you attempt to identify your own fears.

Fear of Feeling Good

You may have already taken the first steps to ending unhealthy eating patterns as you have worked through this program. In fact, you may have done something like this before, and been excited about believing that this time everything's going to change. Unfortunately, you found yourself back to your old patterns and choices all too soon.

Past experience has shown that continuing to do what feels good *to* you and is good *for* you can be extremely difficult. Even now, with the knowledge, awareness, and practice you have under your belt toward changing your eating patterns and food choices, your challenge becomes to continue to focus on your body's messages, respect them, and do what they tell you is best for your body.

Being afraid of feeling good is a common fear. You may have had repeated experiences in your life of enjoying something or somebody and then suddenly having that thing or person disappear, leaving you feeling sad, hurt, angry, and alone. Because these feelings are painful, you may have often become wary of enjoying anything because you automatically anticipate its leaving.

This is the "waiting for the other shoe to drop" syndrome. You anticipate that the good feeling will stop because you will mess up or because someone else will influence you to return to old patterns and choices. You might even believe your disappointment will be more intense the more you enjoy your good feelings now, or that the sadness will be more profound and the loss will be sharper if you feel good about something.

In order to control the timing of the pain you anticipate, you may consciously or unconsciously decide the enjoyment isn't worth not knowing when the good feelings will stop, as you believe they ultimately will. The anticipation of such a loss can produce stress, tension, and anxiety. The fear of not being able to cope with the pain if you don't know when it's coming can block your feelings of enjoyment. In order to protect yourself from something that feels dangerous, you may decide, consciously or unconsciously, that since these good feelings will only lead to pain, you will do whatever it takes to feel bad again in order to break the tension and to control when the pain is going to come.

.Feeling bad, while it doesn't feel good, at least feels comfortable. You can trust feeling bad. You mistrust feeling good. **The fear of feeling good is related to the tension and anticipation associated with its ending**. You may have been taught that nothing good lasts forever. In order to control when the end comes, you choose how and when feeling good will end.

The concept of being comfortable with feeling bad can manifest itself in your life in many ways. You might criticize yourself because you don't do something "perfectly." You might put yourself down every time you make a mistake. You might call yourself names. You might beat yourself up emotionally for just being who you are. Above all, you expect yourself to fail.

Fear of Success and Failure

Many people talk about the fear of success. They blame it for whatever they continue to do that is harmful to themselves. They say they're afraid to succeed because they don't know what success is like, they've never experienced success, or they don't know what to do with it once they are successful.

This isn't quite true. You have been successful at any number of things you have attempted. When you wanted to refrain from eating, you did whatever it took to be successful. When you wanted to eat something harmful, you went out of your way to get it, no matter what the weather or circumstances. You've been successful at hiding and denying eating patterns and food choices you've found shameful for a long time. You've been successful at running away from yourself, at putting up with harmful situations and relationships, and at persevering to make something out of nothing.

That's a lot of success. You know how to be successful, and it's not just successful with harmful issues. You've been successful at learning to drive, at having children, or at getting a job. You've been successful at any number of things during each and every day, including running a household, paying bills, and maintaining relationships, among others.

So, although you think you might be afraid of success, it may be the opposite. You know how to succeed at a great many thing. Therefore, it may not be success you're afraid of, but failure. Failure is painful. Failure has meant something is wrong with you, you're stupid, or that someone will say or do something that will hurt. The fear of failure has often kept you from attempting something at which you're not sure of succeeding. Failure has been something you have probably avoided like the plague because you're afraid of what it says about you.

In order to elude failure, you have become successful at controlling situations where you believe failure is inevitable. In the end, you deliberately fail to take care of yourself because you believe you will ultimately fail at it anyway, and at least this way you can control when it will happen. In other words, you succeed at failing so that the failure happens on your terms. You have been successful at failing.

The fear of failure is a paradox. You fear failure so much that you do whatever you have to do in order to bring it about. This amounts to success. It's not that you fear failing, but you fear not being in control of it when it happens.

The key word here is "when." You believe failure is unavoidable because success would mean doing something "right," and you don't believe you can do it "right," or that you can continue doing it "right." "Right" in this case is translated as "perfectly." It's the belief that you will mess up somewhere along the line which, in your mind, equals failure. In other words, if you mess up, and you already know you will, you will be a failure once again. Mistakes aren't allowed. It's either perfection or nothing.

Because of the tension and anxiety involved in anticipating when this mistake will happen, it becomes much more relaxing to just cause it. In this way, you are in control of deciding when the failure will take place, and you don't have to worry about it anymore. In the end, you're not especially afraid of failing at something, but afraid the failure will come when you're not ready for it. To alleviate this fear, you set up the failure for when you *are* ready for it.

It is not inevitable that you will fail. What is inevitable is that you will make mistakes and you will struggle at times. Contrary to what you may have been taught, however, making mistakes does not automatically mean you have failed. Your mistakes are just one more set of learning tools for you to use. The more you use, the more you have to learn from, and the more progress you will make. As long as you continue to learn, you will never fail.

Fear of Change

Change is something many people fear. The idea of changing your body shape can be especially frightening because of your anticipation of the reactions that might come from others, and your ability to cope with those reactions. This fear of change is usually the result of a twofold belief system at work:

1) The belief that you can't cope with how a change in yourself will cause others to respond to you;

2) The belief that you can control how others might respond by controlling something about yourself.

These are beliefs that stem from the child perspective of being powerless over how you will perceive or react to any new situation (someone's reaction to your new body shape), while at the same time having the power to manipulate the perceptions or reactions of others (no one will say or think anything different if your body shape stays the same).

The first belief is based on the assumption that others will somehow respond in a way you won't be able to manage. If they respond negatively, such as a partner who feels threatened by your new body shape, you may notice your own abandonment or rejection issues causing discomfort. If these issues feel dangerous to you, they may accentuate your feelings of fear to the point that you return to old eating patterns and food choices in order to reassure yourself your relationship will remain as it is.

If they respond positively, such as friends who tell you how great you look, you may become uncomfortable with the thought that others not only notice you but think well of you, or rebel by wondering how awful they thought of you before, and return to old eating patterns and food choices. If you don't subconsciously believe you deserve to have others compliment you, or if you believe there are hidden expectations because of the compliment, listening to others speak positively of your changes may feel dangerous. Your fear of being able to cope is once again emphasized and your tendency will be to return to old patterns and choices.

Relationships are always a major factor to consider when changing. When you continue to view other adults as the people who will dictate the direction of your life and the consequences of your actions, you are looking at them from a child perspective. You remain afraid they will heap negative judgments upon you (and that their judgments are the correct ones), they will cross your boundaries and treat you badly (and you will have to let them or they'll withdraw their love), or they will ask or expect you to do something and you will have no choice but to do it, (even if you don't want to). Staying in this child perspective leaves you feeling as if everyone else is running your life and that you are totally out of control.

It is from this child perspective, then, that you become overwhelmed by fear. In order to dissipate this fear, you will do your best to keep things the same. Even if you don't like it, at least you know what to expect and how to deal with it. You are comfortable with the sameness of your life because you are less afraid of it remaining the same than you are of what change might bring. In other words, even though this part of your life is bad, changing it could make it even worse!

When change happens things *won't* be the same. You will be on unfamiliar ground and the unfamiliar is uncomfortable. Unsure of how the people around you will react and respond, you feel the anxiety and stressful anticipation begin to build. When it becomes more than you believe you are able to cope with, you back down, run away, or return to old, more familiar behaviors. Change becomes something to dread.

It is the fear of change that often generates control issues in people. If you feel you are out of control with your life, you may try to control the lives of others, you may try to control some aspect of your life, (such as weight, food choices, and eating patterns), or you may try to control the environment around you. These control issues are often related to perfectionism. It's at these times that you want everyone in your life to do things your way, you want your body to look a certain way, or you want your house or office to be perfect according to your own (or someone else's) rigid set of standards.

Staying in your adult perspective means the prospect of change, including the loss of what was known and the adjustment to what will come, can be both challenging and exhilarating. As you and your body change, you know that other people may have many different kinds of reactions to your changes, or none at all. You also know you cannot control what those reactions will be. Though you may have a concern about them, you can retain a sense of trust and confidence in your ability to deal with whatever might happen.

It is the reassurance that you will be able to cope with whatever comes along in your life which allows you to welcome change as a part of life. Neither you nor your body are the same now as at seven years old. You have both gone through many changes since then and you have coped with all of them in one way or another. Change will continue and is what provides you with the opportunity for growth. You may retain a certain amount of caution when venturing into a changing situation, but you can remain confident that you can take care of yourself and will keep yourself safe.

This kind of confidence doesn't come about overnight. It takes time, practice, and support from others. One thing you can do to boost your own confidence is to remind yourself of the changes you have already made in your life and to acknowledge that you have muddled through in spite of them. Some of those changes might include getting your driver's license, getting a job, having children, graduating from college, being laid off, starting a class, getting married or divorced, etc.

These are major life changes, and they have encouraged change in you as a person. They meant you would have something new in your life to cope with, whether it was experience, people, a diploma, a title, or a different way to view yourself in the world. Even though such changes may have meant some fear for you, you decided to go ahead with them anyway. You didn't allow the fear to dictate your choice. That is what courage is made of.

Life means change. You have changed physically, mentally, and emotionally since you were an infant. Even though some things were tough in your life, you chose to go ahead with them in spite of the discomfort. You weren't born walking, and you took quite a few falls until you mastered it. You didn't put yourself down or call yourself stupid each time you hit the floor. You persevered until you went beyond walking to running, skipping, and jumping.

It's the same with any change in your life. Walking when you were an infant seemed impossible. However, as you grew stronger, got up, fell down, persevered, and continued practicing, it eventually became easier. Today, unless there are debilitating circumstances, walking is probably as natural to you as blinking your eyes. It's the same for anything new you want to accomplish. You keep at it until you're able to make it happen. This is how you take your power back.

The Fear of What Others Will Think, Say, and Do

Many of your fears probably concern your relationships with others: how they will think about you or judge you, what they will say to you or about you, how they will act toward you, and what they will expect from you. You may be afraid someone will say something negative or judgmental, or that a positive reaction to your changes means they want something from you, including something you really don't want to give. You may be afraid that once someone notices a positive change, they will then expect you to maintain it perfectly. Your changes could simply mean people will notice you in ways they didn't before.

One big fear in relation to the reactions of others is that if your body changes you might become attractive in a sexual way. Sexual attention can be extremely frightening, especially if you have had negative sexual experiences in your past. Often people use the size of their body as a protective device against such attention. People either get too big so no one will find them attractive or too small in order to be as invisible as possible.

Such fears stem from the underlying belief that you won't be able to protect yourself from the pain of other peoples' words or actions, or that you won't be able to stand up for yourself and defend the personal boundaries you have established. This is often caused by a past experience in which you weren't able to protect yourself because you were overwhelmed physically, mentally, or emotionally. The experience happened at a time when you weren't able to take care of yourself and you felt you had no one you could trust to help you. The pain of that experience is something you don't want to go through again.

Because your trust was shattered, you may have developed a mistrust that covers everyone. Your powerlessness in past situations translates into the belief that you can't protect yourself from the pain others will surely inflict on you in the present or future. When you believe you are in danger of being hurt by the reactions of others to the changes in your body, you often experience self-doubt about having the power to cope with those reactions.

As you continually move into an adult perspective and feel your power as an adult, including emotions and attitudes that reassure yourself you are now able to defend your boundaries, you move out of a paralyzing victim stance and into a more cautious adult place of behavior. Give yourself time. Ask for help and support if you need it. These issues don't go away overnight, but they can eventually become manageable and less likely to dictate your choices and behaviors.

Fear of Being Alone

Change in your body shape, food choices, and eating patterns often feel threatening to relationships with the people you feel closest to. If you have had an "eating buddy," whether it's a friend, spouse, partner, etc., that person may now need reassurance that, even though you won't be eating with them in the same ways as before, it doesn't mean you are now judgmental about their way of eating, or that you are looking for a way out of the relationship. Let that person know, however, it *does* mean you will need to find a different way to spend time together and that you would appreciate respect for your new way of eating.

In a couples' relationship that has food and eating as a major source of social togetherness, there will probably be a time of transition so the relationship can be redefined. This is a big fear for people who are part of a "destructive eating" couple. The partner in this relationship may try to sabotage your progress for you by surprising you with your previously "favorite" foods or taking you out to dinner as a "treat." If your partner doesn't stop unhealthy behaviors and attitudes, and you find your focus in jeopardy, you may want to look for outside help. Couples counseling has been effective to not only end the sabotage strategies, but also to help couples find alternatives to eating together as their social outlet.

One reason for sabotage on the part of the partner is their own fear of being alone. They may be afraid that as your body shape changes, along with your personal presentation as your self-confidence escalates, you will want to find someone new. Reassurance for your partner in words and gestures can help alleviate their fears. Even while reassuring them, however, it will be important for you to continue holding your boundaries around unhealthy food choices and eating patterns. If your partner continues sabotage strategies in spite of your reassurance, counseling may be in order.

Fear of Not Getting Enough Attention

One woman I talked to told me she had used gaining weight and dieting as a means to garner attention which made her feel special. She would get a lot of compliments when she was losing weight, but the compliments would stop after she had reached a goal weight and maintained it for a while. In order to reactivate the compliments from others, she would gain weight so she could lose it again.

Everyone needs attention. If people don't get it in positive ways, they will use negative behaviors to ensure the attention keeps coming. Take a look at your own attention issues. If you use food and eating as a way to get the attention you need, you may want to look at the kinds of relationships you're in and how much positive, supportive attention you get from them.

You may be caught up in the "st" syndrome. Being the best, least, most, or worst, biggest, smallest, or baddest at something can make someone feel special, no matter if it's positive or negative. These are the extremes, the all or nothing attitudes that don't allow room for your own individuality because the focus remains on others.

For many people, the idea of living at one extreme or another has been a way of life. In order for you to stay focused on your body and its messages, it is important for you to accept and acknowledge that you don't have to be an "st" person to be happy. Your happiness and self-satisfaction need to come from inside in order for you to continue doing what is healthiest for you. **While acknowledgment from others is important and can enhance your life, your own acknowledgment is what's necessary.**

Fear of Not Being Loved

Making changes in your size and shape can threaten your perception of how attractive you are. If so, you may want to rethink your definition of attractiveness. To do this, it might be helpful to think of someone you thought of as physically attractive, yet as you got to know them personally, and realized you didn't like them as a person, you found them increasingly less attractive. The reverse is true as well. Someone you love may not have a perfect physical shape, yet you find that person very attractive.

There is a reason for this, and that is that physicality is not what ultimately makes a person attractive. Think of the personality traits in people you find attractive. It is their innate sense of being that is attractive or unattractive. It is how they present themselves to the world that renders them attractive.

Usually the most attractive people are those that are warm, open, and willing to listen to and support you whether you're up, down, or in between. They like people and it shows. They have an aura around them that invites you into their world. They let you know you are attractive to them by wanting to be with you.

Your attractiveness is based on the same qualities. How you present yourself to the world goes a long way to rendering you attractive to others. As your body took on a size and shape you didn't like, you may have changed the way you presented yourself to the world. When you feel unattractive, you will usually present yourself in a way that shows it.

For a relationship to be based on more than surface qualities, you have to not only have confidence in your own inner qualities and let them shine through, you also must look for people who value more than physical qualities in their own relationships as well. **If healthy living and healthy relationships are your goals, you will present yourself as such a person and attract, as well as be attractive to, others who feel the same way.** This is not something that is necessarily accomplished overnight, but will take some time, energy, support from others, and risk on your part to make it happen. Again, get help with it when you need it.

Fear of Compliments

A true compliment is a gift someone freely gives to you. It is meant to be enjoyed. It is only one person's opinion, yet it comes from the heart. It may seem ridiculous to think someone could be afraid of compliments, but unfortunately this is often the case.

Compliments often represent personal meaning other than someone giving you a gift they hope you'll enjoy. The way in which you perceive a compliment will determine how you respond to it. If a compliment means you are now in a spotlight, it could be embarrassing. If a compliment means you are now expected to do something in return, it could feel heavy and possibly overwhelming. If a compliment means the person giving the compliment is now going to act differently toward you, it could be frightening. If a compliment means that somehow you have changed, which means the relationship has changed, it could be something to avoid. If a compliment means someone thinks something good about you, and you don't believe you have anything good about you, you will dismiss it as a lie.

Depending on your own experience with compliments and their repercussions in your past, you may be uncomfortable with accepting compliments as simply gifts with no strings attached or expected. If you decide there is a hidden agenda behind a person giving you a compliment, your reaction and response will probably be less than enjoyable.

People give compliments for any of a number of reasons. Their intention will always be their own. If a compliment is being used as a manipulation, you don't have to buy into it. If a compliment is being used as a strategy to get something from you, you don't have to reciprocate. If a compliment is hiding an expectation, you can decide if it's something you want to do or not.

One thing you can always do with a compliment is to simply accept it as something that can feel good and enhance your day. Take the compliment and enjoy the positive aspects of it. If you don't, compliments will probably remain something to be afraid of, and you will respond to them as something dangerous.

These are just some of the more common fears people face that have influenced their food choices and eating patterns. In general, fears are of various types and intensities for each individual. It's unrealistic to expect you will get over all of them at once. Some you may resolve and never be bothered by again. Some will always remain, but at an intensity that no longer dictates how you act. You have the rest of your life to decide which to deal with and when.

Fears and Sabotage

These fears, and any others you discover for yourself, are the means to sabotaging your progress toward healthier eating and living. Fear and sabotage are inextricably linked to your feeling of control, and it is through learning about them and understanding how they work that actually empowers you to do what you need to do in order to maintain your commitment and continue in a healthy, more personally satisfying direction.

Sabotage

According to the dictionary, the word sabotage means an act or process tending to hamper or hurt. Sabotage is the means to obstructing and frustrating the momentum you've gained toward those healthier, more personal choices you've been making.

The quickest way to hurt your progress and to hamper the changes you've begun is to take the focus off your body and its messages. Doing this will catapult you back into unhealthy food and eating choices. It will persuade you to begin eating according to those old impersonal messages that come from outside you. It will generate negative feelings about yourself. By taking the focus off what your body tells you, you will sabotage your progress.

Sabotaging your progress is especially easy to do when your body starts changing its size and shape and you start changing the way you feel about yourself. Sabotage is a response to your fears about changing. Because change is uncomfortable, stressful, and involves the unknown, it means taking a risk. And not only must you take the risk of doing something new, you must also have faith that you can cope with whatever the change brings.

Taking the risk of continuing to feel good about yourself means giving up control as you've known it. When things happen the way you expect them to happen, you feel in control. When you begin new behaviors, you're not sure what will happen. You feel out of control. Sabotage is an attempt to regain a feeling of control because you're more comfortable with old, familiar responses from yourself and others than with this new way of thinking, feeling, and looking.

Sabotaging your progress by returning to unhealthy eating patterns and doing what doesn't feel good for you is an attempt to control the reactions of other people to you and your body. You've probably had a lot of experience with others telling you about the mistakes you've made, heaping guilt on you when you haven't done something perfect, or bringing it to your attention that you've tried and failed before. Even though you haven't liked these responses to your old eating patterns and body shape, they are familiar. They help maintain that negative personal environment you are so used to living within. They feel "normal."

Part of the dynamics occurring in the process of sabotage is the attempt to get things back to "normal." This is where the control comes in. When you are confident about the reactions of other people and your ability to cope with those responses, you once again believe you are in control. This is something you can cope with, and your fear subsides. Sabotage is an attempt to manipulate the reactions of other people so you can feel you are once again in control of the situation and therefore, are able to cope with it.

Even though this is a false sense of control, it helps to make everything feel familiar and comfortable. The danger seems to have passed. The only problem is, in trying to control others, you are once again totally out of control with your eating and hating yourself for it. You then blame it all on yourself for being weak, crazy, that something is wrong with you, etc. When you're feeling miserable for messing it up, you sink deeper into your unhealthy eating patterns. You begin perpetrating that self-destructive cycle you've had so much experience being in the middle of.

Here's an example of how this works: you have been eating in an unhealthy manner for quite a few years, feeling miserable about yourself for not being able to do anything about it. You've heard all the cruel and snide remarks about fat people from childhood on. You believe everyone hates fat people and that fat people are basically lazy, don't take care of themselves, and "isn't it a shame they've let themselves go like that?" You continue to eat, starve, over-exercise or binge and purge.

One day you decide you're going to do something different than the regular diet/lose/eat/gain cycle and you find a program that seems to work for you. You begin feeling better about yourself and your body, you look at the eating process in a new way, and you actually make some changes in what, when, and how much you eat. You like what you're doing and the way you're feeling.

You start getting compliments from others and positive reactions about what you're doing and what a difference it's making. At first this feels great, but something inside that you might not even be aware of starts a worry response: What if I can't continue this? What if what I'm doing doesn't last? After all, nothing like this has ever lasted before. I'll disappoint people. I'll disappoint myself. I'll feel terrible about disappointing everyone. They're all counting on me. They all want me to succeed, but what if I don't? Then how will they feel? I can't stand this!

In order to break the tension that's building and restore your life to what you believe is inevitable, i.e., another failure and disappointment, you sabotage your progress. Because you are afraid that this time won't be any different, that you really can't trust your body's messages, and that everything you've achieved is going to go down the drain anyway, you begin your old eating habits as a way to hasten the process and alleviate the suspense.

Now, even though you hate yourself and the way you're eating once again, at least it feels familiar. You know what to expect from others and from yourself. You believe you have taken control of the situation. You can cope with all this negativity, even if you don't like it. You resign yourself to the belief that things will never change and your life is destined to be miserable. You have sabotaged your progress in order to get things back to "normal."

In order to prevent sabotage before it begins or to stop it once it has begun, it's important to recognize and accept that you will experience a period of anxiety about yourself and others whenever you make changes. Realize that the changes you are making may invite skepticism from yourself and others. This skepticism is very common, but doesn't automatically mean you have to give in to it. When you prepare yourself for the possibility of skepticism, you can acknowledge it if it happens and continue making healthy choices in spite of it.

The Feeling of Power and Control

Power often plays a role when it comes to eating patterns. A big body may be equated with power. If the image of a big man equates to commanding respect because the size of his body is indicative of the power he wields, it may be difficult for him to lose weight. If the image of a big woman equates to being someone to leave alone sexually because she believes fat women are unattractive, it may also be difficult for her to lose weight. These people will often sabotage their progress because of the fear of losing their power.

A small body may be equated with power. Sexual power, business power, entertainment power -- in this case, a person might be afraid to gain weight. Self-esteem and a sense of attractiveness may be completely wrapped around the size and shape of the body. More assumptions are prevalent here. The thinking goes, "Everyone" knows that people only think thin is attractive or sexy. Many life-threatening behaviors, including starvation, drugs, cigarettes, surgical procedures, and excessive/obsessive exercise are a result of these assumptions.

Using your weight as a way to show the world a sense of power doesn't work because a true sense of power comes from within. It doesn't matter how big or small you are; the belief that big/small = power is an image, not a reality. As long as you continue to believe the image, however, you will continue to erect roadblocks to maintaining healthy eating patterns.

Maybe you believe you are truly unattractive. In this case, you will often sabotage your progress because to lose weight runs the risk that someone *will* find you attractive, which will negate your theory about yourself. It may be too uncomfortable to find out you are not as ugly as you believe you are.

You may have had a bad experience when you were thin that triggers fear of a repeat of the experience. Losing weight may be easy, but keeping it off only exacerbates the anxiety that something awful might happen again. In order to alleviate the anxiety, you will put the weight back on.

In all these instances, your perceptions and beliefs play the major role in sabotaging the changes you make in your eating patterns and the weight loss or gain you experience from those changes. These perceptions and beliefs may need to be explored with a therapist in order to get to their core so you are able to understand what they mean for you and your progress. In this way, you can get them to a conscious place of ack-nowledgment and acceptance, which will make it easier to change them. It's through changing your perceptions and beliefs that you are able to maintain the choices you've made.

The Time of Your Life

Learning and practicing how to treat yourself well takes time. Unfortunately, in our "do-it-now" society, we receive a lot of brainwashing to be impatient and to want everything right away. To make changes that stick, however, there are no "quick fixes," no magic pills, and no fantastic diets. You didn't learn how to eat in a non-natural manner overnight -- it took years of receiving messages and actual practice to learn how to be out of touch with your body.

The key to learning anything new and making the changes necessary to implements it in your life is time—time for absorbing new information, time for adjustment to the transition, and time for practicing what you have learned. Giving yourself the time to learn involves a commitment to yourself. You must be the primary focus until what is new becomes part of your routine.

While we all move at our own pace, you have choices as to how fast or slow it is best for you to move. The changes you make now and will make in the future may be more difficult for you than for someone else. Be careful about comparing your progress to that of others. Comparisons can be one of the quickest ways to begin the sabotage process.

This program is part of the learning phase. Referring back to the stick shift analogy, this is where you get your initial instructions about driving and begin becoming familiar with the clutch, gearshift, and where your hands and feet belong. It is the phase that gets you started in the direction you want to go.

The transition phase will have its share of ups and downs. Here is where it will sometimes seem that you are taking one step forward and two steps back. In driving, this is where you begin the actual roadwork. You learn about the car and yourself, how both you and the car respond to various signals, and what to do about each. This is often the most frustrating phase. One of the most important things to remember during this phase is that you will make mistakes and you will backslide at times. Mistakes and backsliding are not indications that there is no hope. They are indications that you are human. When you accept they will happen, it often makes it easier for you to get back on track more quickly.

During the practice phase, there will probably still be mistakes and backsliding, but they will become fewer and farther between. This is the phase in which your new beliefs, perceptions, choices, and patterns become part of your routine. In driving stick shift, this is the phase in which you are experiencing the freedom of actually being able to drive. Your self-confidence is heightened and you're continuing to make choices that are best for you.

There is no right or wrong way to make your way through these phases. You may go back and forth between them. As you learn more about yourself and your body, you may repeat phases, but find yourself at different levels within them. You may think you have all this licked, then find yourself back at the beginning.

What's important to remember is that you will continue to be able to catch yourself more quickly, recognize what's wrong and what needs to be done about it, and make the necessary adjustments. It's an indication of just how far you've come that you are able to identify problems and solutions much faster and with more assurance than in the past.

You Can Have Your Cake and *Not* Eat It, Too

Now is the time to start being picky with just what and how much you eat. The so-called "picky" eaters simply have a more personal sense of what foods they prefer and which foods fit for them. You may find you feel full after eating one grape. That's OK--it just means it's time to stop for now. Listen very carefully to what your body says. You may become hungry again in 30 minutes or not for another four hours. As you listen to your body and start to respect its messages, you may be surprised at what it tells you.

These messages may seem strange, especially at first. They may feel uncomfortable because they're new and different. You may not like your old ways of eating anymore but they are predictable, which gives them a comfortable quality. As you find yourself venturing into the newness of natural eating, the old ways will soon become uncomfortable as well. This new perspective on food and eating may feel rocky and unsteady for a while, but during any transition, adjustments need to be made. This is the time for reassurance. Eventually things will feel smoother.

You may also notice the amounts of food you eat at any one time may vary. Many times you may be eating anywhere from a little to a lot less than before, and you may also occasionally still eat a lot at one sitting. You may still come up against a feeling or a situation where you find yourself stuffing food down, comforting yourself. Remember, there are no judgments here. Talk to yourself, let yourself hear what it is you really need to hear. Allow the adult you are to reassure and comfort the child inside that you will take care of yourself and keep yourself safe. When you aren't able to do this, it's an indication of an issue you probably need some help with.

Elimination

One problem you may have become aware of but don't quite know what to do about is how to manage those areas you have accepted as out of control areas, whether they are food choices, times, or ways of eating. These are the areas when you don't stop eating even though you know you are full, you refrain from eating even when you know it would be important to do so, or you continue to use something in connection with exercise, food choices, or eating patterns to maintain an image instead of exploring and resolving problematic situations.

These are the areas that have resisted every trick in the book and means of willpower or determination known to you. These are the areas that have caused you to believe you're "weak" or that you just "need more self-control." These are also the areas that have contributed to your feelings of shame, guilt, and self-hate.

The reality is, it's not you that is stupid, bad or weak. There's nothing wrong with you. Instead, what may be happening is an addictive process that defies intelligence, strength, or logic. Some theories call addiction a disease, some say it's a learned behavior. No matter what the cause, addiction cannot be controlled by conventional means.

No one can explain the process of addiction in concrete terms. What is known is we aren't able to control it no matter how hard we try. Trying only results in frustration and a sense of failure, as you may have experienced. This is because you've been trying to control the uncontrollable.

As noted earlier, doing the same thing over and over which results in the same, unwanted, unhealthy behavior is a sign that there may be an addictive process at work. If what you've doing isn't working, it's time to do something different. It's time to take true control by giving up the "trying." It's time for elimination.

Elimination is a two-fold process:

1) It acknowledges and accepts that a certain place, pattern, or food is a trigger for non-natural eating.

2) It requires a conscious choice to remove the problem from your life.

By utilizing the concept of elimination, you enable yourself to regain true control over those specific areas which have been problematic for you.

True control means you do something by choice rather than for any other reason. In other words, you are truly in control when you look at options, choose one that is healthiest, and take the action it requires. You choose from a place of personal power instead of from the feeling of being forced to.

Choosing from a place of personal power removes the feelings of "have to's" and "can't's." When you choose to eliminate something from your life because it's not good for you and you admit you can't change what's happening when it's around you, it's not because you "have to" do so or because you "can't" have something anymore. Instead, you choose to eliminate something because **you want to stop hurting yourself**.

When you begin eliminating choices and behaviors from your life because you don't want to hurt yourself with them anymore, you indicate to yourself that you are intrinsically feeling an increased sense of self-worth and self-value. The process of elimination becomes a chance for you to redefine what you want and don't want in your life.

Choices for elimination can include specific foods (some of the more common ones are chocolates, fried or crunchy foods, or sweets), certain places (eating in your favorite chair in the living room or eating at a party), or specific ways of eating (snacking between meals, eating while reading or watching TV, or eating "on the run"). Even though these specifics are distinctive for everybody, the ones that pertain to you will make a significant difference in your attempt at true control.

Elimination is an action. What you choose to eliminate is specific to you. For example, if eating between meals is an area in which you are out of control, snacking would be something for you to eliminate. Other people may be able to eat between meals without hurting themselves, but you can't. Maybe it isn't fair, but it is your reality.

The charting exercise from Chapter III gave you a look at areas in which you personally are out of control with your eating. When you acknowledge your own reality about your inability to control everything, the concept of control becomes something quite different from what you have been taught or have tried in the past.

In effect, when you choose to eliminate a specific food, place to eat or way of eating, you take back the permission you have given yourself to hurt yourself through food. By eliminating something that hurts you, you also give yourself permission to take back your power to define your own eating rules for your life. This in turn eliminates the concept of "cheating" or breaking the "rules."

Your decision is based on what you *want* to do rather than what you believe you *should* do. You eliminate those areas your body has told you are unhealthy for you. As you continue to practice the process of elimination, you finally take true control of your eating.

Through the action of elimination you end the battle you have engaged in every time you are confronted with the food or eating pattern that has triggered out-of-control responses. Instead of trying to use willpower or determination to "only eat one," choosing elimination enables you to automatically claim a victory rather than wallow in a failure. You choose not to take the first one because it's the easiest one to resist. The battle is won before there are any more casualties.

If you have identified some of your out-of-control areas, now might be a good time to do an elimination exercise for yourself. Write down on a piece of paper those foods, ways of eating, and places of eating that are out-of-control areas for you. Next, tear up and toss away those you are ready to eliminate from your life. Say good-bye to those you eliminate. They are no longer a part of your eating life.

Don't worry if you're not able to do any of this right now. Take your time – this process is yours and yours alone. Many find it easier to eliminate something small first, and get used to that change. Some decide they need to eliminate the most destructive item first, and do so. Whatever works for you is the right way for you.

Now that you have gotten rid of the problems, how do you *stay* rid of them? There are various ways and means of helping yourself stay on track with all this:

- Keep in touch with supportive people. You're not expected to do this alone.

- Continue exploring your issues when they are problematic. Remember, as soon as you find yourself eating out of discomfort, there's probably an issue that needs to be resolved.

- Attend support groups, to help keep you on track. If you specifically identify a food/eating addiction, Overeaters Anonymous meetings may be particularly helpful.

- Write about your fears. Seeing them in black and white helps put them into a more realistic light for you.

- Make a contract with another person to call *before* you eat what you really don't want to eat, or before you purge, or as a way to encourage you to eat in a healthy manner. We help ourselves by enlisting the help of others.

- Read your Personal Empowerment Affirmations daily. It's too easy for those old negative, judgmental messages to come crowding back in.

- Be aware of sabotage. Talk to a supportive person about how good you feel about the choices you are making and let yourself wallow in the wonderfulness.

- To see if you've changed anything, go through the first two checklists again to see if anything's different. You may be surprised.

Even if you do all this, it doesn't mean you will never be tempted or have cravings again. Old patterns and habits die hard. New connections with and support from others who can relate to your struggle are extremely helpful in keeping you on track and getting you through the rough spots. In the end, though, your choices are up to you. They make you neither a good or bad person, but simply reflect what you believe is best for you at this time in your life. You'll do what you want when you're ready.

Now you have the awareness, the information, and the tools to make peace with food. You have choices and decisions to make. You have attitudes to cultivate. Your journey is in your hands. It's OK to go at your own pace. Remember that travelling to anywhere takes time. I hope you enjoy your journey and find caring people to share it with. You deserve all the best life has to offer.

To Remember

- Fears are indicators of a perceived danger. Don't ignore them; take control of them by learning about them
- Listen to opinions, explore options, and ultimately choose what you like, want, or what's best for your life
- Watch for indications of sabotage strategies
- Taking your focus off yourself is the quickest way to sabotage your progress
- Taking true control means choosing to do something because it's what you *want* to do
- Mistakes are a natural part of any learning process; be kind, patient, and gentle with yourself
- If one choice continually doesn't work, try something different
- Eliminate that which is out of your control; there is no shame in admitting you can't control everything
- This is your life; you have this body in this life to be responsible for -- no one can do it for you

APPENDIX

PAGE (i)

Where's Your Focus?

_____Something's wrong with me because I can't lose weight and keep it off.

_____I feel like I'm a bad person when I'm fat.

_____I believe others judge me by the way my body looks.

_____I compare my body to others as a way of measuring how I should feel about myself.

_____I've tried different diets, all with the same results.

_____I hate myself for the way I look.

_____I hate myself for the way I eat.

_____I'm ashamed of the way my body looks.

_____I believe the right-sized body will make me feel good about myself, attractive, and/or happy.

_____I believe that only thin is attractive, sexy, or good.

_____If I had more willpower, I wouldn't have an eating/weight problem.

_____I constantly monitor my weight.

_____I am afraid of getting or being fat.

_____I am afraid of being thin.

_____I could always stand to be 5 pounds thinner.

_____If I only lost weight I would/could...

_____I stay thin by non-natural means (fasting, excess exercise, purging).

_____I believe fat is bad.

_____I exercise to lose weight.

_____I would like myself more if I weighed less.

PAGE (ii)

Personal Environment

____I eat when I'm not hungry.

____I don't stop eating when I'm full.

____I worry about eating.

____I worry about not having enough to eat when I'm away from home.

____Sometimes I am afraid to eat.

____I am afraid of being hungry.

____I don't allow myself to be hungry.

____I eat more than I need so that I won't be hungry later.

____I don't eat when I <u>am</u> hungry.

____I restrict the amount or kinds of food I eat because of guilt feelings.

____I "binge."

____I sneak or hide food.

____I don't know how to tell if I'm hungry or not.

____I don't always know why I eat.

____I am ashamed of what I eat.

____I eat what I "shouldn't."

____I don't eat what I "should."

____I don't stop eating until I'm stuffed.

____I don't know how to tell when I'm pleasantly full.

____I feel out of control with my eating.

PAGE (iii)

Picture Your Body

PAGE (iv)

Picture Your Emotions

PAGE (v)

Describe Your Body

PAGE (vi)

Technology and Consumerism Manipulation

2019 excerpt from an interview with Douglas Rushkoff, author of *Team Human.* Interviewer is Sean Illing.

Douglas Rushkoff

In a more practical sense, the way it works with individuals is you go on a platform like Facebook, and Facebook is using data from your past to dump you into a statistical bucket. Once they know what bucket you're in, they do everything to keep you in that bucket and to make you behave in ways that are more consistent with all the things about that bucket.

So if they know there's an 80 percent chance you'll go on a diet next month based on your search habits, then they'll start peppering your newsfeed with articles and stories that are designed to get you to really go on that diet. You'll see stories of people getting too fat or whatever. And that's to get you to behave more consistently with your statistical profile.

Sean Illing

The algorithm thing is tricky to me. On the one hand, algorithms are making our lives easier by predicting what we want and giving it to us. On the other hand, our wants are so manipulated, so curated, that at some point it's no longer a meaningful choice and the algorithms are just doing our thinking for us.

Douglas Rushkoff

And what if you don't want anything at all? That's the thing: That's not one of the choices you have online. So in that sense, they're not even giving us what we want. They're trying to trigger whatever they can *get us* to want. It's about stoking consumption, about convincing us that we need another gadget, another toy, another device that will make us happy.

Sean Illing

And part of your argument is that these forces are turning us into atoms of consumption and consequently eroding our connections to other people.

Douglas Rushkoff

Right, and again, the roots of this go back way before digital technology emerged. TV and consumer advertising wants us to be unsatisfied and disconnected from other people so that we look to products to fill that void. And products can never fill that void, which is great for the marketer, because then we'll keep buying stuff to fill an ever-expanding void.

PAGE (vii)

OLD MESSAGES

- Food
- Eating
- Body Image
- Expectations
- Numbers
- Reward/Punishment
- Guilt/Shame/Blame
- Judgments
- Should/Shouldn't
- Comparisons
- Perfection
- Bad/Good

TROUBLESHOOTING

Date	Reason for Eating	Did/Didn't Stop	Meaning for Food

PAGE (ix)

DISCOMFORT WITH EMOTIONS
TOUCH—INTIMACY

Date	Emotion Touch Intimacy	Reassurance	Praise

165

PAGE (x)

CHILD/ADULT PERSPECTIVE

Issues	Child	FEAR GAP	Adult
Dependency/ Survival Ability	Dependent on others. Abandonment. Rejection. Co-dependency issues.	⇒	Inter-independent. Connected to others. Can take care of self.
Perspective/ Knowledge/ Experience	Narrow—Few Options Fantasy—All or Nothing	⇒	Reality-Based Options, Opinions. Gray Areas
Time Comprehension Discomfort	Now or Never Quick-Fix Fear and Danger	⇒	Patience Caution Assessment

Focus Individuation	Comparisons/Denial Self as related to others	⟹	Listens to, trusts self. I am OK.
Self-Worth Self-Value	What do I matter? Non-assertive, passive	⟹	Sense of personal Know boundaries, self
Personal Empowerment	Little power/ Blaming Tell me what to do	⟹	Empowered Responsible for actions

CHILD/ADULT CHART

Date	Problem/ Solution	Quick- fix	Appropriate Coping	Reassurance

About the Author

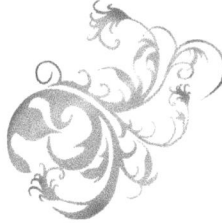

Sandra Yelich, MSW, has worked in the field of addictive and other harmful life patterns since 1982. She has studied Brief Family Therapy, EMDR trauma therapy, and relapse prevention. She has also created and facilitated groups in areas including relationships, team building, and trust issues, assisting group members in recognizing self-destructive behaviors and identifying positive alternatives.

Sandra created the program **How To Make Peace With Food** in 1993.

For any questions or feedback, feel free to reach out to Sandra at slsfelipe@yahoo.com

www.ingramcontent.com/pod-product-compliance
Lightning Source LLC
Chambersburg PA
CBHW020256030426
42336CB00010B/784